Copyright © 2018 by Geoffrey Cooling. All rights reserved worldwide. No part of this publication may be replicated, redistributed, or given away in any form without the prior written consent of the author/publisher or the terms relayed to you herein.

Geoffrey Cooling, Hearing Aid Know, 4 Stratton Audley, Bicester, Oxfordshire, OX27 9AU, United Kingdom

If you would like to contact me to ask a question, please don't hesitate to send an email to info@hearingaidknow.com.

Table of Contents

The Introduction To The Little Book	3
Let's Talk Providers of Hearing Aids	5
Big Corporates	6
Independent Hearing Healthcare	9
Online Hearing Aid Sales	12
What You Need To Think About When Buying A Hearing Aid	18
What Happens at The Hearing Test	26
Bring Someone To The Test	34
Choosing The Right Hearing Aids	38
Fitting and Following Up	42
The Advent of Telecare	46
Understanding Hearing Aid Pricing	49
Hearing Aid Manufacturers	54
Widex	55
Phonak	60
Starkey	69
Signia	72
GN Resound	77
Hearing Aid Types	80
Receiver in Canal Hearing Aids	83
In The Ear Hearing Aids	87
Behind The Ear Hearing Aids	95
Wireless Hearing Aids, Bluetooth Hearing Aids, What's The Difference?	98

Rechargeable Hearing Aids	100
Hearing Aid Technology	110
Hearing Aid Features, What Do They Do?	117
Over The Counter Hearing Aids, What Will They Mean	128
Cleaning & Caring For Your Hearing Aids	134
In Finishing	141

The Introduction To The Little Book

Welcome To The Little Book

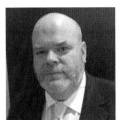

This is now the third edition of the Little Book, over the last few years; I have expanded the content in response to feedback from people who have bought it.

I regularly correspond with buyers of the book and I thoroughly enjoy the feedback. I wrote this book originally because I wanted to make sure that there was a good, impartial source of information available to people.

It is exactly the same reason I got involved with the website Hearing Aid Know. In this book, I have again updated the information given and expanded it to include some of the latest developments.

My background is relatively simple, I have been involved with hearing aids for over ten years and they continue to fascinate me. I was a qualified hearing aid dispenser in private practice, before moving to work for a major hearing aid manufacturer. I am now back in private practice, operating in Dublin Ireland.

As I said, I collaborate with a guy named Steve Claridge on the website, Hearing Aid Know. We want to bring clear honest advice to consumers centred on hearing aids and the people who provide them. I like to talk straight, laugh at gobshites (Irish technical term) and my sense of humour may well get on top of me.

However, bear with me and I am usually able to translate the gobbledygook. Privately provided hearing aids are a big investment, I want to give you the knowledge to make that investment with confidence.

What follows is a relatively high-level look at hearing aids, their technology levels, their pros and cons and the features inside. I hope that this will give you the complete grounding in the subject that you need to make educated decisions. In one review of this book, it was said that I don't do a comparison of hearing aid brands.

I don't, it would make the book about a thousand pages long. All I will say is that each of the major hearing aid brands offers relatively outstanding hearing aids that do what they are supposed to. I like Phonak hearing aids, however, I was wearing GN Resound LiNX 3D 9 hearing aids up to recently (loved them, blew me away). I am currently in love with Signia Pure 312 Nx hearing aids (stunned almost to silence by the own voice processing) and a set of Oticon Opn 1s (very different to anything I have ever tried but I love them).

I see my job in this book to give you a high-level understanding of what should actually matter to you. I also try to make sure I at least touch on the latest and best hearing aids from the major manufacturers. Without actually physically seeing you, I can't do a comparison and recommend the best for you. It is just impossible.

In one of the reviews given for one of the books somebody said I was encouraging people to go to Audiologists. In the UK and Ireland we don't have the same set up as in the US. We are all Hearing Aid Audiologists. There are no Hearing Instrument Specialists and Doctors of Audiology here. So while I might have mentioned Audiologists in the text, it wasn't meant to be a recommendation to see an Audiologist in the states.

My feeling in general would be go to the person who has excellent reviews, no matter what their level of qualification. In my experience, I have seen Hearing Aid Audiologists, Hearing Instrument Dispensers and Doctors of Audiology who were halfwits who I wouldn't let treat my dog. So level of education is no guarantee of efficacy.

I would ask you a great favour, if you are happy with the information this book arms you with, I would ask that you review it on Amazon. Your reviews give prospective buyers the confidence to buy the book. Thank you in advance.

You can read more about hearing aids and the people who provide them on our website at Hearing Aid Know

Let's Talk Providers of Hearing Aids

Providers of Hearing Aids

In the UK and Ireland, you can access public healthcare to get hearing aids. I know the US is different for the general public, but Veterans can also access a form of public healthcare through the VA.

The hearing aids available through these schemes are actually pretty damn good. The service generally isn't. The reason is simple, the services are underfunded and the clinicians who work in them are usually under serious pressure.

That is the way of the world though when it comes to public services. I don't cover the hearing aids available or the service provided by public healthcare in this book. I concentrate on private healthcare and private provision of hearing aids.

In order to privately procure a hearing aid you need to attend a provider, pretty simple really, however, you have a choice of different types of providers available to you. That choice has grown in recent years beyond the two traditional outlet types.

There are corporate type providers such as Amplifon, Hidden Hearing, Boots and Specsavers in the UK and Miracle-Ear, Hear USA and Beltone in the US.

There are also Independent providers who may be large multiple branch outlets or smaller single outlet businesses.

In the recent past, we have seen another type of provider arrive, the Online Provider. They offer savings based on the fact that they have no shop front and small overheads.

In the next few pages, I would like to explore these outlet types and explain the pros and cons of each one of these very different provider types.

Big Corporates

Corporate Providers

Corporate providers generally offer a pretty good service including on-going aftercare, although with many it can be a bit like a conveyor belt. I worked for Amplifon in Ireland back in the day and I have to say that they were on the cutting edge of best practice and service. We provided an outstanding level of service to our Patients and they still do.

However, we worked within the constraints that were set and our business was sales, don't get me wrong, it also involved real committed care, but sales were what it was all about. Most corporate providers are built on this system, there is always some pressure on staff to sell, which is simply how they survive.

Pressure To Sell Specific Products

There will usually be some pressure on staff to sell one product line specifically in most corporate chains. Again, Amplifon were a little different, they have a wide selection of brands but the pricing of the devices tends to control what is sold. Amplifon is a corporate entity but it is, in fact, independent of any manufacturer. That allows them to make decisions on product sales which are more based on market demands than hearing aid manufacturers needs.

Arrangements with Manufacturers

Amplifon have arrangements with particular manufacturers and those arrangements mean that certain brands are more advantageous for them to sell. However, as long as I was there, Corporate Management didn't interfere at the macro level. They simply allowed Dispensers sell whatever they felt was best for the Patient in front of them. I always found that admirable.

Owned By Hearing Aid Manufacturers

Many corporate providers are in fact owned by hearing aid manufacturers. While some of them may have different hearing aid brands on their price lists, they are more likely to sell you the brand that owns them. The fact that a business is owned or part-owned by a hearing aid brand is very rarely obvious or publicised.

For instance, Boots in the UK is owned by Sonova, the owners of the Phonak and Unitron hearing aid brands. In the US, Sonova owns Connect Hearing. Hidden Hearing (another UK company) is owned by William Demant, the owners of the Oticon Brand.

Beltone in the US is owned by GN Resound. It just isn't these hearing aid brands; every major hearing aid brand has some sort of retail arm. This type of vertical integration is just increasing within the business, more and more manufacturers are buying retail outlets.

Limiting of Choice?

I believe that this vertical integration limits your choices, the equation is simple, and more often than not you are getting one brand no matter what. Honestly, this doesn't necessarily mean that the device or brand won't be suitable for you; it just means there is no real choice on offer.

I honestly don't think that this is necessarily a bad thing; I just think that you should be clear on it. They really should make it clear to you; I believe an educated decision is nearly always a good one.

In essence, while corporates try to ensure that the best service and experience is on offer across their chains, it is sometimes not the case. Another problem with Corporates is that there can be a good bit of staff turnover, so you may buy from one person, but end up being seen by another at a later date.

I know that some people find that off-putting, they like to stay with the person they trust, especially if they have built up a relationship with them. However, the fact that Corporates have multiple branches and staff can also be a pro.

If for instance, you are travelling in the UK or across the US, if your provider has an outlet wherever you are, they will see you as a customer if you get in trouble with your hearing aids.

It is also worth considering that if you have issues with the person who supplied you with the hearing aids, there are also other staff members to take care of you. These things do happen and I personally have seen them happen many times.

So there are pros and cons to dealing with a corporate entity, just as there are pros and cons to everything.

Independent Hearing Healthcare

Independents

Independent providers are just that, local independent businesses who are independent of any hearing aid manufacturer or corporate entity. They are usually small family run single Practice businesses, although some may be multi-branch. More often than not though, they are single branch entities that may offer their service in branch and perhaps across a few clinics situated in associated health partners such as Opticians or even Chemists/Pharmacies/Medical Centres.

Access to All Products

Independents generally have access to all of the big hearing aid manufacturers, however, in practice, they will usually only use perhaps three brands at most. There will be a primary brand that they deal with and two secondary brands. Generally, these are picked for a variety of reasons, some commercial in nature such as pricing and some clinical in nature such as efficacy and perhaps specialisation.

I have said before, that if I was running my own Independent practice I would probably choose Widex, Phonak and GN Resound as my three suppliers, however, that decision has got harder for me. Since I said that, both Oticon and Signia have introduced technology that really interests me.

So my choice would be a little harder now. I would try to choose the brands that were able to provide me with pretty much everything I needed to meet the needs of my customers as they presented to me.

However, as different innovations came along I would be considering other brands or re-considering what share of each brand I supplied. Let me explain my thinking, Phonak is recognised as the leader in power hearing aids, so I would always consider Phonak for my power needs, however, GN Resound is the one manufacturer who offers outstanding and versatile made for iPhone power hearing aid.

So it makes perfect sense for me to discuss these brands with someone who needs a power aid. Widex has a Power offering called the Super, but it is several years old now so I would discount it because I believe that both Phonak and Resound have superseded it with better technology.

Independent hearing healthcare professionals are often the very first to receive access to new technology. For the manufacturers, they are the most profitable channel so it makes sense for them to ensure Independents introduce everything first.

In line with this, Independents are often some of the best trained professionals. Or at least, they are nearly always the first to get the training. All of this, gives Independents freedom.

Freedom to Offer Best Service

That is the freedom that total independence delivers, you make the best decisions based on the customer in front of you and the latest and best technology available. I think that is the best way to serve the customer, and indeed, the best option for the customer.

Local Business

Most Independents are local businesses, they often live local to the community they serve. That is the way business used to be done; you did your business with someone from your locality, which meant that the money was in general kept in your locality. More than that though, you knew who you were doing business with. You might not have known them personally but there was always word of mouth through the community.

Service Instead of Advertising Budget

Independent businesses tend not to have massive marketing budgets. Their success is generally built on service and good word of mouth. They don't survive unless there are both. Independent professionals usually rely on the word of mouth of their customers to succeed in business. The simple fact is that if they don't treat people right, they don't eat. That has to be seen as a pretty big incentive. However, more often than not, they are genuinely caring and committed to offering the very best service.

Often Higher Levels of Care

Independent hearing aid providers offer high levels of service and aftercare as standard. Normally they have set up their own businesses in order that they can do just that. National hearing aid providers are getting better and better at looking after their customers, however, everything within those providers is usually to a rigid plan.

Independents are truly flexible in their approach, delivering the service and aftercare that is needed when it is needed. You probably won't find many others who are as committed to ensuring you have the best experience. On top of that commitment and because a hearing aid provider is Independent, he or she does not have to march to the company guidelines when it comes to providing hearing aids.

It simply means that they will recommend hearing aids that are right for you and your lifestyle needs. Hearing healthcare professionals in National businesses will always try to do the same but because of company policies and changing commercial arrangements, they may have to do so within a limited choice.

Online Hearing Aid Sales

Online Hearing Aid Retailers
In recent years there has been an explosion in online hearing aid providers. Initially, the online providers were in fact, little more than lead generation sites. Their only business was to get your name and address and sell it on to a business local to you. While that model still exists, there has been a divergence in the space in the recent past.

Buying a Hearing Aid Online
The sales of hearing devices online are not new, there are businesses around the world that sell hearing aids online direct to consumers. In fact, some of those businesses do an excellent job of it, in the main because they have that infrastructure in place to ensure the buyer's success. That infrastructure involves remote testing of the buyer's hearing and remote fitting and fine tuning of the devices.

However, that is not the case with all online hearing aid retailers. Some of the new online retailers are offering hearing aids from the big hearing aid brands, hearing aids that were never designed to be sold online. Let's talk about online retailers. There are now three types of online hearing aid retailers, they are

Lead Generation Sites

Co-operative Groups

Hearing Aid Retailers

The lead generation sites don't really need much description, they are simply there to attract you to them, get your name and address and then sell it on to someone in your area. They have in fact been around for years and they are leeches. They use their skills to get enquiries that they sell to hearing aid providers. There really isn't much else to say about them. The others are a little interesting and work differently.

Co-Operative Groups

Co-operative groups have essentially spawned from the lead generation sites. They are in essence a group of hearing aid businesses (usually Independents) who are co-operating to drive a website which brings in enquiries and business.

There is a centralised control of the website and enquiries are sent to the nearest hearing healthcare professional in your area. From my own point of view, I find these sites more palatable because at the very least they are run to help Independent hearing aid providers to thrive.

Hearing Aid Retailers

There are now several true online hearing aid retailers, some of them such as Blamey & Saunders or Eargo manufacture their own hearing aids and sell them online to the public. Some, however, sell hearing aids from the big six hearing aid brands. These types of business usually do not have a network of Audiologists that they work with, although, that is beginning to change.

I don't think online sales of hearing aids are a bad thing when there is an infrastructure set up to cater for it. By that, we mean that the online sales are supported by a testing and fitting infrastructure either online or offline.

For instance, Blamey and Saunders in Australia deliver a system I would support as does iHear and Eargo in the US. These companies have purposely set themselves up and designed their technology to be delivered online. The support and infrastructure to deliver it are clearly there.

However, I would not support the sale of hearing aids from the big brands that are not really designed to be sold in that manner. The underlying technology to do this well with the main hearing aid manufacturers just really isn't there right this minute.

That doesn't mean it won't be in the future but right now to look after someone remotely is difficult at best. You need to be aware of that when you are making a decision. I am not saying it is impossible, however, it is difficult. Later in the book I will discuss Telecare which may well change this situation.

What You Need To Know When Buying Online

So here it is, this is what you need to consider when buying online, and the first and most important thing is that hearing aids are not like glasses. You don't just put them on and everything is wonderful. It simply doesn't work like that, unfortunately. You will need care and attention to get the very best out of your hearing aids for as long as you have them. That may well be between eight to ten years. If you feel confident that the online retailer can give you that care and service and is committed to doing so, then you are onto a winner.

It is both my experience and the experience of Steve that to get on well with hearing aids people generally need the involvement of a good hearing healthcare professional. We have said it here before, our worry about buying hearing aids online was that people may buy the hearing devices and then find it difficult to get a professional to help them. This is a worry in particular from any site selling hearing devices from the major hearing aid brands because again, they are not really set up for remote care. So there are several things you really need to consider so you can make an educated choice before buying.

What You Need To Think About When Buying a Hearing Aid Online

- Hearing aids aren't glasses, they don't just work
- You will need ongoing care
- Will someone give you a professional and in-depth hearing test?
- How will you understand what are the best hearing aids for you?
- Will someone make a recommendation on the best hearing aids for you?
- Will someone fit them for you?
- How much will the hearing test and fitting cost?
- How much will it cost for aftercare visits? (you are going to need them)
- How much will it cost for repairs to be handled?
- Finally and the big one, will the extra costs of getting someone local to help you mean a net saving or loss for you?

It struck me that the question I should answer is "Would I be happy to sell you hearing aids online?" That is the real test, isn't it? So I should answer it, I would be happy to sell you a hearing aid online if, and it's a big if, the hearing aid manufacturers made the technology available that allowed me to do an in-depth hearing test. Allowed me to do a full fitting and verification of the hearing aids and finally and probably most importantly, that I was confident that you were able and tech savvy. Right now, those conditions don't exist, so No, I wouldn't sell you a hearing aid from one of the big manufacturers online right now.

What does it Matter to You?

First of all, you want the latest and best for you and your hearing loss; it is as simple as that. Secondly, hearing aids aren't the same as glasses. You do not just put them on and everything is fine. That is a simple truth, hearing aids take time to get used to, and they also take time to get the very best out of. This is usually called rehabilitation.

You might not realise it but the services of a good hearing professional are absolutely imperative to your ongoing experience. In order for you to get the best out of any hearing aids you buy; you will need a committed and skilful professional to help you.

Of course, those are all pros, but what about the cons to dealing with Independents? If it is basically a one-man show, there could be issues with continuity of service. God forbid he or she gets sick, is injured or dies, who will continue to look after you?

If you have issues with your devices while you are travelling, will you have access to help? In fact, that depends, if the issue is with the failure of your hearing aid, then you will probably be able to get it fixed under your warranty elsewhere.

Your International Warranty will cover you for such repairs during the warranty period. However, there may well be a handling charge for it. After all, you aren't a customer of the Practice that is organizing the repair and post and packaging needs to be covered.

For anything else, such as diagnosis of issues, adjustments, wax traps, batteries etc. You will have to pay or negotiate a local price.

Why do You Need Help?

As I said, hearing aids are not like glasses; firstly, by the time you choose to buy hearing aids, you will probably have been suffering a hearing loss for up to seven years or more.

If I was to give you full amplification (the prescription you needed to correct your hearing), you would run screaming from my office. You wouldn't like it one bit, you would find the level of amplification overwhelming.

So, I will first set you to a reduced prescription, one that benefits you but doesn't challenge you too much. You will still note a dramatic difference, however, it will be as much as you can handle. Over a period of time that really does vary from customer to customer I will then increase the amplification to your prescription level.

Not every Professional will follow this protocol. Modern hearing aids have an auto-acclimatization feature. It is a feature that I can set, at the first fitting which will gently turn the hearing aid prescription up towards your prescription level over a controllable and customizable level of time.

I use the system; however, I still like to see the customer during this period to assess the increase and to discuss the changes and their experiences. I believe that this is the best way to serve my customers.

The prescription that is used is based on your individual hearing loss. The prescription is based on thousands of hours of research and thousands of ears. It is an excellent starting point, however, everyone is different. I have found that most people need further personalization of their prescription to get the best out of their hearing aids.

So, with that in mind, even when you get to your prescription level, you still need some tweaking. I think this makes the situation a bit clearer, and it is why you can't compare hearing aids to glasses, or perhaps any other device. Let's talk about customization of sound.

Think it's Over Then? Think Again

Like I said, the prescription isn't when the fat lady sings, generally, your prescription level is just a starting point, a good starting point but just a starting point. Hearing is a very personal sense, and appreciation of sound differs. I like classical music my wife thinks it is noise. Each one of us is slightly different, unique in a way. Most people will need some fine tuning undertaken around their prescription to be happy with the sound of their hearing aids.

So finally, after all those appointments we have got you to a place where the sound the hearing aids produce is just right for you. That's when we start investigating the settings for different situations and discussing how you are getting on generally. This just doesn't happen in the first week or month, this takes time and effort both on your part and the part of the professional who is helping you. That professional needs to be dedicated to helping you.

What You Need To Think About When Buying A Hearing Aid

Buying a Hearing Aid
Purchasing a hearing device is a big decision on many levels; firstly there is a big financial outlay involved. On top of that is the psychology that seems to be inherent in the decision. It never fails to surprise me, the deep thoughts and stigma around hearing aids, but you aren't old, it isn't a sign of you losing it, it simply is. Let's take a look at the psychology of it.

The Lies We Tell Ourselves
Hearing loss just happens; the best thing to do is deal with it. I wrote on the Hearing Aid Know site about the lies we tell ourselves about why we don't need hearing aids and I want to detail them here.

My Hearing Loss isn't Severe Enough
Hell no! Your wife or husband is about to strangle your ass. If she or he has to repeat themselves one more time she (it's usually a long suffering she by the way) or he will happily kick you until your unconscious!

Even a Mild Hearing Loss
Apart from all of that, even a mild hearing loss needs to be treated. In fact, recent evidence that has come to light in relation to untreated hearing loss and cognitive decline frightened me so much I started wearing my hearing aids all the time.

Hearing Loss & Cognitive Decline

Let me explain, we as professionals were always worried about the wider effect of hearing loss on general health and emotional well-being. In the last few years though, evidence has come to light that connects untreated hearing loss to more rapid cognitive decline and possibly dementia.

In essence, we are now sure that untreated hearing loss causes more rapid cognitive decline. The evidence points towards this increased cognitive decline contributing to dementia. Are we sure? Pretty much so, but there is still an elusive part of the puzzle to be found.

The evidence has made us as professionals change our own thoughts about intervention in hearing loss. We are now recommending hearing aids even for mild hearing losses that we may not have before.

So, it's pretty simple, if you have a hearing loss at all, you should really think about treating it with hearing aids if they are appropriate.

Hearing Aids are Uncomfortable

Yes, that's right; they are strange at the beginning. You have never worn something in your ear all day before. Why in hell would they not be uncomfortable or foreign? That feeling will fade with a little time. If it hasn't faded within a week you may need to be re-sized, generally, it is a simple process.

Stop using excuses because you don't like the idea of wearing hearing aids. Time to get over yourself, which brings us onto.

I would be Embarrassed to Wear a Hearing Aid

So, I understand that actually, I don't feel it, but I do understand it. For me it is a simple equation, need hearing aids, gets them. I really don't give a toss what other people think, in fact, I am probably famous for it. But, I do understand that other people don't see it as that simple for them. They see having to wear a hearing aid as some sort of statement about them, the ageing process and their worth.

Truly, is it more embarrassing to be in control of your own ability to communicate or to stumble through life trying to bluff something while everyone knows you have a problem?

That's all arse (Irish technical term) complete and utter arse. A hearing loss is not a statement on you, on who you are, on how old you are, it simply is. No more and no less. It is a problem that is causing you real issues. Not doing something about a hearing loss that is affecting your life is a statement about you.

Truly, is it more embarrassing to be in control of your own ability to communicate or to stumble through life trying to bluff something while everyone knows you have a problem? Because believe me, everyone knows you have a problem.

Exactly What You Are Missing

Let's think about this, what are you missing, what are you losing out on by not dealing with your hearing loss? The whispered words of a loved one, the simple joy of a particularly moving piece of music, the words of your Grandchildren, the joy of easy social contact.

So much of the joys of life are based on communication and engagement. Robbing yourself of the ability to be truly involved is just damn stupid. Are you stupid? I don't think you are, you bought this book right? But let's make it clear, life is supposed to be lived, and a major part of that is the connection to the people and activities that you love.

Get your hearing aids and get on with it.

The Joy of Easy Communication

How much do you miss the joy of easy communication, getting the joke first time, instead of them having to repeat themselves? The frustration of having to ask someone "what did they say?" The sitting in a room of people you love while being almost completely isolated. The simple joy of easy conversation.

You know the next time you are tired and worn out from the effort needed to just listen? You know that feeling of stress, that feeling of being overwhelmed? You know the simmering strife in your home life because the people you love are at their wits end? Well, most of that can be easily dealt with by using hearing aids.

Damn it, Reclaim Your Life!

Reclaim your life, it is as simple as that, are you ready to pack up and die? Well if you aren't, get on with living.

I do not want to admit a hearing loss in public

Why? I go back to my last statement; everyone knows you have a hearing loss. Believe me; they knew long before you really did. So what are you really worried about? You are worried about being embarrassed, but believe me and you know it well. You will be more embarrassed by getting everything wrong, asking people to repeat themselves and generally looking like you are doddering a bit.

Yup, doddering! Let me ask you this, which looks older and a little senile? A person who seems to be constantly forgetful, who asks others several times to repeat themselves, gives the wrong answers to questions, constantly confuses words and constantly goes on about how people didn't mumble so much in my day.

Or, someone who takes control of their ability to communicate lives an active social life and is generally happier with their lives? Think about that, I know what the right answer is and so do you.

Hearing Aids Do Not Work in Noisy Environments

Yes, they do, especially if you buy the right level of technology for you. Simply put, if you want to hear well in complex sound situations you need to think about the top two levels of technology. Does that mean that the bottom two levels of technology won't help you?

No, it doesn't, they will help you a great deal, especially if you use something like a remote mic to give you an extra bit of help. Hearing aids will work to give you the sound cues you need to understand what is being said. Will they allow you to hear everything in a really noisy situation? Maybe not, but you have to realise that even people with perfect hearing have problems with noise sometimes.

The key to being happy with your hearing aid purchase is to be realistic about what you should hear with them. You need to be realistic about your expectations of the hearing aids you buy as well. A good professional should guide you on this, they should try to make it clear what the hearing aids can be expected to deliver.

I Have More Serious Priorities
Actually, you probably don't, back to what I was talking about earlier. Our new understanding of the effects of hearing loss on general health and cognitive function makes treating hearing loss a priority. As I said, we have changed how we think and we are recommending the treatment of even mild hearing loss.

I do understand that there may be other things going on in your life, things that make it difficult to consider your ability to hear as a priority for you. But your ability to hear is your ability to communicate with ease. That has an effect on all the different parts of your life.

They don't Restore Your Hearing to Normal
I am afraid nothing can restore your hearing to normal, but hearing aids do a damn good job at giving you normal levels of hearing. They are the difference between hearing what is being said and saying what? All the time. They will allow you to communicate freely and easily.

I Hear Well Enough in Most Situations
Yes, about that, nope. Ask your long-suffering family about that. One of the things I hear often is that I hear well in one to one situations. Generally, people with hearing loss do okay in one to one situations where their companion is facing them and the face is well lit. With no competing noise and full view of the person's face, they get on okay.

However, we do a simple speech test with many people, words presented at normal speech levels. Of course, there are no visual references so they are relying on the hearing only. When they have gotten three out of five or six out of ten words wrong, they suddenly realise they aren't doing as well as they thought they were.

Damn it be a grown up
Yup, enough prevaricating, enough lying to yourself, enough excuses. You owe it to yourself and your ongoing health and happiness. Hell, you owe it to your long-suffering family. Time to put your big boy or big girl pants on. This is too important to hide behind

bull, believe me when I say it. Hearing loss isn't a statement of who you are, not getting proper treatment for it and trying to bluff is.

The Price is Important, But so are Other Factors

Many first time buyers focus on the price of the instruments, I can understand that because they tend to be expensive. There are many other factors that you need to consider when you are thinking about buying hearing aids.

But let's focus on the price for a minute; generally, the price of a hearing aid includes a lot of services, in fact, years of it. For years I have spoken about unbundling prices so it is clearer exactly what you are paying for, not many have done it. I believe that will probably change though as pressure to justify cost increases.

The price of hearing aids I charge to you is based on a simple calculation:

Hearing aid cost + (How much my time is worth x how much time I spend with you) = Hearing Aid Price

I will go into the price considerations in a deeper manner later, but here I want to give a quick overview and talk about White Label hearing aids.

Hearing aid price breakdown

An understanding of the price structure is important, so what are you paying for? Generally and certainly in the UK and Ireland, you are paying for the hearing instrument itself and all of the care and support that you are expected to be given for the lifetime of the instrument.

All of the private hearing aid dispensers in the UK and Ireland offer a similar service. Professionals in the US generally offer exactly the same thing. You need to be clear on what is on offer to you though.

Because with that knowledge, you can make an educated decision. The general Patient Journey that is on offer is as follows:

The fitting of the hearing aid

Follow up fine tuning visits to ensure the aid is customised for you (perhaps two or three). These are exceptionally important visits and during this time the basis for the success of your hearing aids is set.

Either six monthly or yearly follow up appointments to service the aid and ensure you are still doing fine from then on. During these visits you can expect to have your ears checked, the hearing aids checked and at least once a year your hearing checked.

Lifetime of a Hearing Aid

You may hear it said that the lifetime of a hearing aid is four to five years, that's not true. Generally when people talk like that, what they actually mean is that the lifetime of hearing aid technology is four to five years. By that, I mean that innovation in the hearing aid world tends to move in four-year cycles. Every four to five years something new comes out that is truly extraordinary in comparison to what went before.

The lifetime of a hearing aid, however, can be up to about ten years, after eight it can become difficult to get it repaired if it fails. So during that period, you are going to attend a lot of half hour to hour sessions with your hearing professional for re-testing-fine-tuning and aftercare.

That is exactly what you are paying for, time and professional expertise. When you have paid for it, don't be embarrassed about taking it up. I think that my time is worth money, just like any other professional who offers service, when you have paid me for that time; I always make sure that you get it.

Going For the Cheapest Price?

There can be a disparity in prices across different providers and it can be attractive to simply go for the cheapest option. What you have to ask yourself is, "is it like for like?" This is the most important question that you need to ask yourself; later in the hearing aid section, I discuss hearing aids and their technology levels. I do so in order that you can consider this question in a more educated manner.

The cheapest price is not always the best option; you need to know all the facts surrounding that price and the equipment and service offered before you can make an educated decision. What service will be offered, what exactly are the hearing aids, are they the latest technology? When you have answers to these questions, it is easier to make decisions.

White Label Hearing Aids

Some corporate providers offer white label hearing aids, white label hearing aids are devices made by manufacturers with a special label. For instance, Specsavers has the Advance range, Hidden Hearing has their own range which is made by Oticon, in the US Costco has the Kirkland range which was made by Resound and is now made by Signia. Starkey does its own white label for its retailers.

I personally don't like white label ranges, I understand the commercial reason why they are used but it makes them hard to analyse for the consumer. That is exactly why a white label is used, to make it difficult to do like for like comparison. It is easy for a Dispenser to say oh they are the same as such and such, more often than not, they aren't.

They may be made by the same manufacturer but how are you to know exactly what they are? The information is never really forthcoming, maybe it is my natural sense of suspicion, but why do they need to hide the brand name in the first place?

So there is a lot of information to take in when you are buying a hearing aid and it is easy to feel overwhelmed by the sheer amount of information that you need to consider. That information is both medical and technical in nature, medical when it comes to your hearing loss and technical when you are trying to understand any hearing aid technology that has been recommended.

There is a lot of choice in both types of hearing aid available, and the manufacturers who make them. It can be quite difficult for a consumer to understand it all and sort through what is important. A good Dispenser will help you on that journey, deciphering the gobbledygook. Before we move onto hearing aids and their technology, I want to take a look at the experience of buying a hearing aid, what should happen and why.

What Happens at The Hearing Test

The Hearing Test

The quality and comprehensiveness of the hearing test is important. You should get a complete hearing test undertaken by a qualified professional. Our understanding of your ability to hear is built up through many different tests. The benefit delivered of different test procedures like speech audiometry and speech in noise testing to the eventual fit of a hearing aid was once debatable.

However, with recent changes in hearing aids and our own understanding of hearing loss the more in-depth the test is, the better the recommendation and eventual fit. Information derived from speech testing and speech in noise testing, in particular, is very valuable in understanding which hearing aid is best for you.

This information can also be incorporated into the fitting of the hearing aid delivering a better personalisation for you. Ideally, audiological tests should be done in a soundproof booth for complete accuracy, or at a stretch a very quiet room. Although with the advent of new types of audiometers designed to eliminate outside noise that is actually beginning to change.

The consultation should also incorporate more than just testing procedures. To understand your hearing needs, a hearing health professional should discuss your medical history, lifestyle needs and the issues you are having. After the test is finished the professional should explain to you the severity of your hearing loss and what type of loss it is.

At this point, they should be able to recommend to you which kind of hearing aids and which technology level will work best for you, your lifestyle needs and your loss. Let's take a look at the hearing test and the different processes.

The hearing test appointment will usually last between one and one and a half hour. The test is made up of several different overall parts that allow a professional to understand the full background to any hearing loss, any medical issues pertaining to your hearing and then your ability to hear.

Each part of the process is designed to furnish different information that is then used to make recommendations. Each part of the process has a certain value and will shape the recommendations made. After the hearing test is complete, the professional will explain clearly what he or she has found and will make recommendations on those findings.

What happens during the hearing test?

Generally, the hearing test no matter where you get it will follow the same pattern with similar components. Components within the overall parts may differ based on who is providing the test and the results they are getting. For instance, some professionals may not undertake speech in noise tests at all, and middle ear testing may not be undertaken unless something points to it being specifically required. Having said all of that, the hearing test will usually include:

Examination of the ear and auditory canal, including video otoscopy

Case history

Full audiometric hearing assessment that will include pure tone testing, middle ear testing and possibly speech testing in quiet and noise.

Explanation and discussion of outcome

Impartial advice on the most suited hearing system for your individual requirements

Let's talk about those stages in more depth.

Otoscopy (Examination of the ear)

This part of the assessment is about the health of your ear, your outer ear and your ear canal. The professional will first examine the outside of your ear using a light. They are looking for any blemishes strange marks or sore spots. They will then use an instrument called an otoscope to examine your ear canal and your tympanic membrane (eardrum).

This again is to check the health of your canal and eardrum. They will check something called the light response on the eardrum; this is simply the way the light is reflected on the drum. A healthy tympanic membrane will reflect the light in a specific way. This examination may also give indications of problems with your middle ear and indications of any history of perforations.

It also allows a professional to become a little familiar with your ear canal. Each ear canal is different, different sizes, different bends. Once the professional is happy, they will move onto the next part.

Case History

A case history is taken to get an understanding of the background of your hearing loss. During the case history, you will be asked typical questions such as your name, address and date of birth. They will ask you about any treatments in the past that may have used ototoxic drugs (medicines that are toxic and damage hearing).

Then the professional will ask you questions about any background to the hearing loss, such as your working history when you noted an issue if the issue occurred suddenly, has it worsened suddenly, do you have tinnitus, if so is it in only one ear etc.

These last few questions are designed to allow the professional to assess if you have what is called a referrable condition. If they find this to be so, they may well continue the test but will refer you on for further examination by an ENT professional. Once this is done the professional will also ask you questions about the perception that you have of the impact of your problem on your daily life.

These questions are important because it allows the professional to begin to understand your lifestyle and the impact if any that hearing loss is having on it. Sometimes these questions may seem odd, but to get a good understanding of what is best for you, we need to have a good idea of who you are and what you enjoy doing. After the case history is undertaken, they will move onto the auditory testing proper.

Auditory Testing

Auditory testing is made up of several tests that assess the full function of your auditory system. It is important that the testing is comprehensive, but certain parts of the test may not be needed depending on results from earlier tests.

What happens during auditory testing?

As we said, not all tests may be undertaken, for instance, masking and middle ear analysis may not be needed, however, best practice auditory testing involves the following tests;

Pure tone testing (audiometry)

Masking (audiometry)

Speech in quiet testing

Speech in noise testing

Tympanometry

Acoustic Reflex Threshold testing

Distortion Product Otoacoustic Emissions (DPOAE) testing

Audiometry (Hearing Test)

Audiometry or pure tone testing is a series of tests where pure tones (sound like whistles and chirps) or warble tones (similar but they oscillate or vary) are presented through a set of headphones, insert earphones or a bone conduction headband. It is important that both air conduction (through headphones) and bone conduction (through bone conduction headband) are both undertaken.

Air conduction audiometry tells us what you can hear from the outside in; bone conduction audiometry tells us what your best inner ear can hear in isolation. This is important because sometimes there can be a difference and this is the clearest method to identify if you have either sensorineural or conductive hearing loss or indeed a mixture of both.

The results are plotted on an audiogram which shows your hearing sensitivity in the tested frequencies. These tests tell us the softest sound that you can hear and allows us to tell you if your hearing sensitivity is within the normal range or if there is a hearing loss.

Audiometry results tell us many things beyond just your hearing sensitivity; it allows us to see if there is any asymmetry in your hearing loss (a hearing sensitivity that is not equal between the two ears). It also allows us to see the configuration of your hearing loss (the shape of the way your hearing loss occurs tell us a lot about your hearing loss causes). This and other tests can help towards a diagnosis of ear abnormalities.

How is audiometry performed?

The initial test involves you carefully listening through headphones (air conduction) that are placed over the ears or insert earphones that are placed in the ear canals. Pure tones will be presented with the headphones or insert earphones. This part of the test is called air conduction testing and is designed to allow the professional to assess what you can hear from the outer ear.

If you hear the sound, you will push a button or raise your hand in response. The professional will continuously reduce the volume of the sound until you can no longer hear it. The key here is that the professional is trying to identify the softest sound you can hear, so no matter how soft it is if you think you hear it you should push the button. Many people are never sure and feel like they are letting down the professional.

This couldn't be further than the truth, just relax and don't get frustrated. Once the headphone or earphone test is undertaken, the professional will then change to a bone conduction vibrator on a headband that is placed behind the ear or sometimes in the middle of your forehead. This part of the test is designed to find out what your inner ear can hear, it is very rarely different but in cases of conductive hearing loss, there will be a marked difference.

This part of the test is important; a previously unidentified conductive hearing loss is a referrable condition. Even if you know that you have a conductive hearing loss and it has been assessed by an ENT, the results are still important for the programming of any hearing aids that may be prescribed.

This overall test will determine your hearing thresholds and would normally be the end of the audiometry testing. However, just occasionally the results will point us to undertake advanced audiometry. This is where we earn our money!

Additional tests called masking may be added to the group of tests if an asymmetry of thresholds is found or if you have a conductive hearing loss. Masking is very important and there are clear rules when a professional needs to do it. Masking is designed to keep one ear busy, while the other is tested. In essence, it is only undertaken where we do not trust our original results.

As I said, there are clear rules on when we should mask and when we should not trust results. You will know masking because the professional will play a white noise type sound in one ear which they will tell you to ignore while they ask you to respond to the normal beeps or whistles in the other.

Speech Testing

Words will be presented at a comfortable listening level either free field which is presented through a calibrated speaker or through headphones. You will have to repeat the words and the professional will score you on the results. This test gives the professional a deeper understanding of how you hear speech; it also identifies the speech sounds you are missing.

The test will then be undertaken with increasing levels of background noise. This test is an important part of the assessment, it will give the professional a lot of information about how you perceive speech and the signal to noise ratio you need to hear and understand speech in noise.

These types of tests have always been done; however, in the last few years' speech in noise tests have become more helpful to us. A test like Quick SIN allows us to understand the signal to noise ratio that you will need to hear speech well in noise.

Why is it important?

The level of sound you hear is only a starting point for our understanding of the impact of your hearing loss. This just tells us the mechanics of the sound levels. Speech testing actually allows us to understand how well the brain centres that manage hearing are working.

It is often the case that speech scores can be radically different between two people, even if the audiogram results are the same. The speech in noise testing also allows us to understand exactly what type of hearing aid technology level is most suitable for your hearing loss. For best diagnosis and hearing aid recommendation, the Quick SIN testing protocol has become a must.

How is speech testing performed?

Most independent hearing health professionals have updated their testing equipment to allow them to run automated speech and speech in noise tests through their audiometer. During these tests, you will be asked to repeat words that are presented to you at normal speech volume levels with and without noise.

Word recognition scores will be determined and recorded on their system. The Quick SIN test will give a signal to noise ratio score which will give a professional a clear idea about the hearing devices that will help you in noise.

Middle Ear Analysis

What is middle ear analysis?

Middle ear analysis tests are undertaken to assess the function of the middle ear. The tests will assess how sound travels through your middle ear and also how your brain reacts to some sounds. You will feel a short blocked sensation while a recording takes place.

These tests are not necessarily important; they only become important if there is a clear need for them. So if I have identified that there is some sort of mid ear issue, Tympanometry will help me understand what that issue might be?

Tympanometry itself will not have any bearing on the hearing aid that is fitted, the audiometric results will. There are two parts to the Middle Ear Assessment: Tympanometry and Acoustic Reflexes.

Tympanometry

What is tympanometry?
It consists of measuring how much your eardrums are moving and if that movement is within normal limits. It tells us if there is any fluid or congestion behind the eardrums. (Presence of fluid behind one's eardrums is known as glue ear, and it is very common in children).

This test measures how well your middle ear works. Your middle ear includes your eardrum, the middle ear bones, and your Eustachian tube. It will reveal abnormalities which will signify and can explain a conductive hearing loss and/or a sensation of pressure in the ear.

How is tympanometry performed?
An ear tip is placed in the canal that is connected to a handheld machine; it briefly varies the pressure in the ear. By varying the pressure, the movement of the eardrum can be measured. It takes only a few minutes to complete. You will not need to respond to this test.

Acoustic Reflex Thresholds

What is acoustic reflex threshold testing?
When we hear a loud noise, our ear protects itself with a reflex which stiffens the eardrum. We use this reflex to test the Facial and Auditory nerves. This test measures how the stapedius muscle contracts in response to a loud sound. The absence or presence of acoustic reflexes can be important for differential diagnosis.

How is acoustic reflex threshold testing performed?

Often, tympanometry and acoustic reflex thresholds are done together. With the ear tip in your canal, you will hear beeps that are progressively louder. You will not need to respond. Instead, the machine will automatically measure the response.

Distortion Product Oto-acoustic Emissions (DPOAE)

What is DPOAE testing?

This test measures how well the outer hair cells in the cochlear work. The outer hair cells produce low-level sounds called Otoacoustic Emissions in response to clicks. A conductive or sensorineural hearing loss will often result in absent DPOAE responses.

How is DPOAE testing performed?

With an ear tip in the canal, clicks are presented in the ear. In response, the cochlear emits a sound which is recorded by the equipment. The extent of the response and the frequency at which the response occurs is measured and recorded.

Explanation of the results

Once the testing is complete, the professional will explain the results, they will explain exactly what they have found and detail why it is having the impact it is in your life. They will also make recommendations based on their results in order for you to return to a more normal level of hearing and allow you to engage fully in your life.

Hearing Aid Benefit Assessment

If you are a suitable candidate for hearing aids, many professionals will then move onto a hearing aid benefit assessment or demonstration. In essence, what they will do is programme up a set of demo hearing aids to your loss, they will not give you full amplification but a level close to it.

This will allow you a taste of what hearing aids sound like and how they will work. Any professional worth their salt will move through a demonstration of different features explaining to you as they go what they are and how they will work for you.

Bring Someone To The Test

Go to the Test Accompanied
You should always take a loved one with you to your hearing test; firstly, undergoing any kind of medical examination or procedure can be stressful. It is always a good idea to take someone with you to a medical appointment. Whilst caught up in the process and worrying about results, it is easy to miss other important information. If you have someone with you they can help to remember what was said. It is always better to have two people in order that as much information as possible is retained.

On this point, feel free to make notes during the appointment and don't be nervous about asking questions. Query anything that you do not fully understand. Conversely, don't be afraid to ask the Audiologist to write something down for you. A true professional will not be put out by being asked questions; these questions will come up, it is better to ask them at the appointment. As a professional, we understand that this experience is new to you and the information is foreign. We also understand it is our job to help you understand. It is also important to have your family involved in the process.

Hearing Loss is a Family Sport
Hearing loss affects every member of the family, not just the person who suffers from it. Communication is a problem, often frustrations creep in. Family members may feel that the person with hearing loss is in denial or just ignoring the impact of the hearing loss. If the person with hearing loss has withdrawn from their social circle, family members may be concerned about their well-being. Hearing loss tends to have an effect on the entire family.

Denial is Not Just a River in Egypt
A great old Dublin saying, "De Nile is not just a river in Egypt", usually uttered as someone shakes their head and throws their eyes to heaven. There is a lot of talk about

denial in hearing loss and there is certainly an element of denial involved in many cases. However, denial is fed by a misunderstanding of how hearing loss works.

Cultural Understanding of Hearing Loss

Firstly, most people really don't understand how acquired hearing loss works or how it will affect someone's ability to hear. Most of our understanding of hearing loss is formed by TV, Radio and Theatre. In that world hearing loss is not just something to laugh at, it appears to be all about raising the volume. "Speak Up, Speak UP, What Did You Say?" It is all very Monty Pythonesque.

Hearing Loss is rarely about Pure Volume

Run of the mill acquired hearing loss is very rarely about volume, it is nearly always about balance in sound. In fact, hearing loss that is about pure brute force volume is quite rare and it is usually something that is present from or related to something from, birth. In normal, run of the mill acquired hearing loss, there is an imbalance in the ability to hear sounds. Some sounds can be heard quite well or even normally, while other sounds may not be heard at all.

I Can Hear The Voice!

Quite often, someone with hearing loss can hear someone's voice very clearly; they just can't really understand what some of the words are. If you think about that for a minute, you can see why it is easy to think that the problem is, in fact, the speaker, not the listener, if they can hear the voice, surely the problem is that the speaker isn't speaking clearly enough?

The actual problem is that more often than not, someone with hearing loss can't hear consonants in speech. So basically words sound indistinct and mumbled. The person isn't mumbling you just can't hear them properly. However, you can see why it is easy to think that the problem is the speaker rather than your own. That is in fact why people take so long to realise they are having problems. It is also why they are loath to release the idea that it isn't them, it's everyone else.

Helping You Make a Realisation

When family members attend a hearing test, they will often help their loved one towards a realisation in relation to their hearing ability. It is the family who really understands the effect of hearing loss on the person who has it. They see and understand when there are problems, in a clearer manner than the person who is suffering them. Don't forget, as a person with hearing loss, you don't miss what you have missed. Or to put it another way, you don't know what you don't hear.

People around you do. While you may be unsure about the depth of the problems you are having, the people around you tend to see them clearly. I have often witnessed a Patient come to a clear realization of their problems simply through the testament of a family member. Quite often, it is the first time that the discussion about their hearing loss is undertaken in a clear and focused manner.

More often than not, it also leads to the sharing of worries that have been unsaid. Concern that has often been unvoiced.

Keeping You Honest

The other thing that a family member will often do is to keep you honest. I have spoken here and on the Hearing Aid Know site about not fooling yourself. As I said, family members tend to see what is really happening and generally aren't afraid to give you the unvarnished truth. Nor are they afraid to speak up when you are lying to yourself. They have a way of telling you how it is. I find the reaction to hearing loss a very strange thing; it seems to be one of the few health issues that are surrounded by personal stigma.

Hearing loss is not a statement about you, it just is!

People will outright lie to themselves about their ability to hear in order to protect themselves from the thoughts in their heads! It never fails to surprise me, I have said it before, and I have no doubt I will say it again, hearing loss is not a statement about you, it just is.

Helping Them Understand

Your family doesn't really understand hearing loss any more than you do. Attending the appointment will also allow them to understand the issues. It will also allow them to become familiar with your hearing loss and the effects it has on your ability to communicate. The hearing test will make it very clear to them exactly what the issues are and why you have the problems you do.

Moving Forward

If you move forward with hearing aids, the involvement of your family with your ongoing rehabilitation plan is important. They need to understand the advantages and limitations of the hearing aids you have chosen. They also need to understand how they can help you, especially during the early stages of rehabilitation.

A Better Understanding of Progress

As you move forward with hearing aids, family members can also help to assess your progress. They can also help identify areas where you are still having issues with your hearing. I love when family members are involved in the process; they are a secondary source of information which allows a full picture of what is going on. They are also a validation of the problems. Let me explain that.

When someone has an issue hearing they automatically think it is their hearing loss and the fault of the hearing aids. Sometimes, it isn't. There have been times where a Patient has spoken about problems with a particular situation or a particular person. The family member has chimed in and said, I hadn't a clue what they were saying either! Or I couldn't really make it out with all the noise going on either. In essence, if they can't hear, neither should the Patient be able to.

In contrast to that, some Patients may think they are doing pretty well in some situations and the family member may be able to point out where there are some deficiencies. All in all, the inclusion of the family in the process has to be seen as a good thing for both the Patient and for them. So get your family involved early.

Choosing The Right Hearing Aids

The Hearing Aids

If a set of hearing instruments is recommended to you, don't be afraid to ask the professional to write the details down for you if you wish to research them. As I said some companies may offer white label instruments, these are instruments that are re-named by the manufacturers specifically for the company you are dealing with. If you are being offered something like that, ask exactly what the instrument is based on and from what manufacturer.

Don't be nervous about asking questions; ask about the different kinds of hearing aid available which are suitable for your type of hearing loss. Ask why the particular hearing aids have been recommended. As I said, a professional will not be put off by any questions. Don't be afraid to say that you would like to research the hearing aids that have been recommended to you.

On Hearing Aid Know we try to offer a decent high-level view of most hearing aids to give a good understanding of what they will do for you. My friend Abram Bailey runs a website called Hearing Tracker, it can be found at

www.hearingtracker.com

The site offers rundowns of both hearing providers and hearing aids in the US; it also has consumer reviews of both. It is a pretty good place to get an idea about the effectiveness of both the hearing aids and the providers who are listed.

Hearing Aids, Have Realistic Expectations

You need to have realistic expectations of the hearing aid technology you buy and what it can deliver for you. Modern hearing aids are exceptional pieces of technology, but they are not, nor probably will never be, a replacement for normal hearing.

The higher the technology levels of the hearing aid, the better the results for you. Keep this clearly in mind when you are making any purchase decision. Don't buy low technology hearing aids and expect them to help you in all situations, they simply won't.

Knowing What You Want Helps

Before you decide what to buy, have a clear idea of what you want from your hearing aids. Think carefully about your problem situations, consider where solving those problems are important for you. If you keep that clear you can consider what type of technology level will be best for you.

If you have a sedentary lifestyle and all you want hearing aids for is listening to TV and Radio, some light conversation and the occasional journey to the shop. Low-end technology should almost certainly meet all your needs.

However, if you have a busier lifestyle and your hearing aids will be imperative for more complex sound situations, then higher levels of technology are most certainly for you. Key to any decision is the understanding of your needs and realistic expectations of the technology level of hearing aids that you will buy.

With this in mind, you will know what you can expect from what you can afford. When this is clear to you, it will make your journey with your hearing aids less stressful for you. It is the Dispenser's job to make this clear to you and they often will, however, you need to really listen.

It isn't a sales technique, they aren't trying to up-sell you, and more often than not they are simply giving the best advice possible. It is up to you to decide what you get within your budget, just be clear about what that will deliver to you.

Wireless Accessories

In recent years most hearing aid manufacturers have moved towards wireless communication within their hearing aids. This connectivity has opened up new options and resulted in new accessory devices that deliver real benefits for hearing aid users. There are many additional extras that can now be purchased with your hearing aids. These are all useful add-ons which can help someone with hearing loss to lead the life that they are used to.

I really think that these devices are outstanding, however, as with many things; they are only useful if you actually are going to use them. Each manufacturer will offer some wireless solution, the question is do you need them? These can increase the costs so think carefully before buying. Don't pay for something which you might not use very often or pay for something you don't really need.

However, having said that, if you are constrained by your budget, and you can't go for the technology level of hearing aids you would like. An accessory can help to make up for what you are missing. For instance, a wireless remote microphone can really deliver fantastic results for hearing in noise even when paired with a low technology hearing aid. Keep this in mind when you are making the buying decision.

Be Sure Of What Are You Buying

So you have made the decision to buy, you have picked out the aids and the accessory you want. You need to be sure about what you are actually buying. Ask the seller to explain in detail what you are actually buying, if they say lifetime aftercare, ask exactly what does that mean?

The life of the hearing aid, a set period of time, your lifetime? What does that aftercare include, are there structured callbacks, will you drop back when you have a problem, or alternatively will they just call you for a re-test in five years?

These are all things that you really need to know, I have said it before, hearing aids are complex devices that need care and attention to deliver to their best ability. Hearing problems are not like vision problems, hearing aids are not like glasses, you don't put them on and everything will be fine.

You need support and rehabilitation and that support needs to be ongoing. So it is important that you clearly understand what you are buying when you pay your money. What aftercare and help will you get?

General Considerations

When choosing the size and shape of an aid, an important consideration is your dexterity. You may find that smaller hearing aids are difficult for you to handle and insert. Not just that, the battery that powers it, may be too small for you to handle, if your eyesight is not great, you may also have issues with the size of the aid or the battery.

Always remember, you are a customer as well as a Patient and if you feel that you want to try something different or go away and think about it, then do so. I have mentioned aftercare already, but it is imperative that you understand what you are buying.

Find out about aftercare and warranty servicing of your hearing aids. They are an expensive investment and you should always check exactly what is included in the warranty and aftercare service.

Make Sure You Have a Written Agreement

Finally, make sure you have a written agreement, then you always have a reference to the agreement you have made. I sincerely hope that this advice will allow you to make educated hearing healthcare decisions. Find a company that you feel comfortable with, ask them lots of questions about the hearing aids that they offer, what they think would be best for you and what exactly is their service offering and you should never go wrong.

Better Hearing, an organisation in the States offers an excellent rundown on buying hearing aids. It can be found here:

http://www.betterhearing.org/hearingpedia/hearing-aids/guide-buying-hearing-aids

Fitting and Following Up

Fitting the Hearing Aids

So we have covered the hearing test and making your decision about buying hearing aids. Let's talk about the initial fit of the hearing aids and the aftercare. Firstly let's look at the actual fitting of your new hearing aid devices, what do you need to consider and what information should be given to you?

The Fitting

The fitting itself is usually a relatively short exercise; the professional will place the hearing aids on and programme them to your hearing loss. We would undertake some tests in relation to how you are hearing and verify that they are delivering against the targets that have been set. The initial prescription level we set will often not be the optimum prescription. This is in order that the hearing aids do not overwhelm you. You will need to acclimatise to them and this will happen over time.

However, we would programme the hearing aids to automatically increase the prescription gently to move you towards the optimum prescription over a period of time. This is called automatic acclimatisation and it is something that is done slowly, in fact, you will barely notice that the amplification is changing as you wear them.

Getting Comfortable With Your Hearing Aids

We will always try to ensure that you are fully comfortable with your hearing aids. When we say comfortable, we don't just mean physically. You need to be comfortable not just wearing your hearing aids but also handling them. In relation to physical comfort, you will be wearing your hearing aids every day, all day. Initially, they will feel odd, in particular, if you are a first time user. However, that should settle down very quickly.

We will make sure that you are able to insert the hearing aids in, or on, your ears by yourself. We will also ensure that you can take them out with ease. It is important that you can handle your hearing aids with ease and confidence; otherwise, they will not fulfil their purpose as solutions to deliver you a better life.

The Batteries

We will show you what batteries you need and how to put the batteries into your hearing aid. It is important that we assess that you can manage the batteries by yourself. We will make sure that you can both handle them and put them in by yourself, we will also give you information on where you can buy batteries, how much they cost, and why it is a good idea to keep spare batteries handy.

Controls on Your Hearing Aids

If your hearing aids have any controls, we will show you how to use them and what they do. You should make sure that you can operate all of the hearing aid controls yourself, and change the listening programmes if in fact there is any. It is important that we assess whether you have the dexterity to operate the controls for your hearing aid. If your hearing aid is supplied with a remote we will show you how to use it.

At the initial fitting your professional may not actually enable the controls or add extra sound situation programmes. Sound situation programmes are excellent tools for a hearing aid user. For instance, a dedicated Music programme is an ideal solution for someone who likes music.

What is good for speech recognition, is not great for music enjoyment. So having a special programme dedicated to handling music is a boon. There are other sound situation programmes that I have found very useful for users. However, and in general, I don't do anything with them at the beginning.

The first fitting and the period following it until the first follow up, is just about getting the hearing aids in, changing the batteries and getting used to the sound.

Cleaning & Caring For Your Hearing Aids

We will also show you how to clean and care for your hearing aid. At the first fitting, we will tend to gloss over these things. Again, we don't want to overwhelm a user with information. However, during the follow up appointments we will go over cleaning and care in a more in-depth manner.

Hearing aids are a big investment, taking good care of them makes real financial sense. We will talk about keeping earwax out of the sound bore and changing wax guards if your hearing aid has them. We will also talk about daily cleaning routines and why you should use a dehumidifier box as part of your care routine.

Proper care and maintenance of your hearing aid are important, it will ensure that it continues to help you hear better for longer. At the initial fitting, all of this will just be a quick run through; we don't want to overload you with information. We will ask you to read the owner's manual and at further appointments, we will ensure that we reinforce the information and that you can clean and care for the devices.

Assistive Listening and Alerting Devices

A hearing aid may not be the whole answer for you, in certain cases, there may be some assistive devices that make sense for you and your lifestyle. Most hearing aid manufacturers have released their own wireless devices for hearing aids.

However, there are many more available from non-hearing aid manufacturers like smoke detectors and amplified phones. We will always give you information regarding assistive listening technology such as the telecoil, mobile phone technology, how best to use phones etc. Again, most decent professional will reinforce this information several times over several visits.

The Follow-up Visit

Your first follow up visit is an important time for you and us. We will begin to detail in-depth cleaning and care, we will begin to start the discussion around sound situation programmes. We will also start to assess how you are doing with the hearing aids and address any issues you have.

We want to know how you have been doing and how the hearing devices worked for you. We will ask you about your listening experiences with the devices and how you have been wearing them. You should be prepared to give us an update on how you have got on in all the different listening situations you have been in.

The questions we ask will cover how you did in noise, your perception of loudness, clarity, any discomfort, etc. Tell us everything, we really want to know, we want to know how you got on. It is worthwhile for you to keep a notebook or diary during the early period so that you can keep track of how you are getting on. This can be invaluable for us because the information is written down as it happens.

Fine Tuning

It is not unusual for fine tuning of your hearing aids to be needed, as I said, sound is a very personal sense, think of music. To one person rock is sweet music indeed, but to another, it is a racket. In the same manner, what is right for one person with hearing loss may often be wrong for others. During this time you will also become accustomed to the hearing aids, this takes some time. Again, the time it takes differs from one to the other.

It may also take some time for you to get the best out of your hearing devices. While we restore normal levels of hearing, it takes the processing centres of the brain some time to adjust. It takes time for your brain to sort out this new sound information. This period is called the rehabilitation period, while initial improvements happen quickly, full rehabilitation can take up to a year.

Reinforcement of Information

As I said, at this visit, we will also take the opportunity to reinforce all of the information we have already given you. We will again discuss the hearing aids and their functions and talk about your clean and care routine.

Ask Your Questions

You will probably have many questions of your own at this stage, make sure you ask them. We have given you a large amount of information during your earlier visits. If any of it is still unclear to you, ask us to go over it again. Since your fitting, you may have new questions. We try our best to cover all of the information you need to know and to make sure you understand.

However, even we forget things from time to time, so ask any questions and that you think you need an answer to. If you need it written down, ask us to do that as well.

The Advent of Telecare

Telecare

Telecare or remote care has been something that has been discussed within our profession for a long time. It offers the opportunity to reach remote Patients, offering them the care they need without travelling long distances to be present.

Traditional ideas of telecare are being explored across the world in areas where populations are dispersed and access to hearing healthcare is spotty. However, hearing aid manufacturers have turned their attention to the concept to deliver better service to the people who wear their hearing aids. Their latest moves may change the way we look after hearing aid users for ever.

Introduction of Telecare by Signia

The introduction of telecare by Signia was an interesting development. In essence, Signia introduced a system whereby your hearing professional could make limited fine-tuning changes to your hearing aids remotely through an iPhone app that was connected to your hearing aids. I liked the concept a lot although many within the Profession were a little suspicious. As with many things within hearing aids, once somebody had done it, it wasn't long before someone else decided to improve it.

Expansion of Telecare by Resound

Resound went one step further with the launch of their 3D platform. They, in fact, offered complete remote fine tuning capability to the Professional, again through an iPhone enabled app. I thought to myself, now you are talking. However, I still felt there were elements missing and I expected the functionality to increase. Obviously Signia have been reading my mail.

Complete Real-Time Telecare

Signia, not to be outdone, expanded their telecare offering to offer complete fine-tuning ability and incorporated the ability to make voice calls to the Professional within their telecare app. But they didn't stop there.

Face to Face Remote Meetings

They have also incorporated video calling to the system which means that Patients can now have a remote, face to face meeting with their professionals for aftercare and fine-tuning.

Why Should You Care?

I think that telecare will evolve and every hearing aid brand will offer their own flavour of it. In fact, Starkey have just announced as we were going to press that they are introducing hearing aids this year which will have a telecare function. Again though, it will not be something that every hearing aid user will be interested in. But I believe that as hearing aid user demographics change, so will the uptake of telecare.

What it Will Do

Simply put telecare will make life easier for users and professionals alike. It will mean that a hearing aid user will not have to attend the office physically to have changes made. It will also mean that Professionals can vary their follow up schedule. Perhaps including one or two remote sessions into the schedule.

Moving forward and as the technology changes and evolves it could open up a different business model. I mean what if the hearing aid brands made remote fitting possible? That could mean that the online business model would be more effective than it is now. It could also mean a complete change to how we as Professionals work.

Complete Remote Care

For instance, how would you feel about a future where you bought hearing aids online and where fitted and cared for remotely by a call centre in anywhere? I certainly don't think that would be palatable for everyone, but I can imagine there are some who would be happy with that if the price were right.

Telecare will continue to evolve and how we do business will do so as well. The biggest influence on what happens will of course be you. The consumer will demand and we as a profession and an industry will need to respond. I see the place of telecare in what I do and what I offer, however, I would hate for it to completely replace the face to face meetings I have with my Patients.

Many of which I have become close to over time, Patients tend to become like an extended family. Some you love, some that irritate you, but all of which you feel a connection to. At least that is how it works for me.

Understanding Hearing Aid Pricing

Hearing Aid Pricing

In the first edition of this book, I stayed away from hearing aid pricing, mainly because it made no real sense to talk about it because it varied dramatically across the world. I still am not going to speak about individual prices here, because I simply don't know what they are. However, I am going to try and explain in detail how my pricing is reached and why it might differ dramatically across organisations.

On Hearing Aid Know we try and include price guides for the UK, Ireland and the US. They are aggregate price guides just giving ballpark prices that we have been able to discover. If you are interested in one particular hearing aid and its price in your country, you could have a look on Know to see if we have listed it. Really what I want to do in this book is to explain how we come to the prices that we do.

What Goes Into The Price?

The retail cost of a hearing aid is based on similar factors across every organisation. The cost of the device to the retailer, the cost of delivering the device to you plus profit. It is a relatively simple equation or matrix. If you were to just judge the cost of hearing aids at a retail level against the cost at the wholesale level you would consider the difference extortionate.

However, it isn't a simple mark up, you aren't just buying a product. You are buying a product and a level of service which includes multiple visits. That service is supplied by a professional who sets a price on his or her time and experience. I am one of those professionals; I think my time, experience and knack for making hearing aids dance is worth money.

Let's break down the price

Cost of devices (varies by technology level obviously and by any agreed discount levels)

The hearing test itself which is at least one hour (in the UK and Ireland this is often free, but if you buy the hearing aids it is kind of bundled into the price)

The fitting of the hearing aids, an appointment which usually takes at least forty-five minutes if not more.

Initial follow up visits, I like to do at least two during the first month. If at the second follow up visit I am not happy with the progress, I will schedule at least one more for two weeks later.

Ongoing service calls, there is some debate about how often this should happen, many feel calling you back once a year is enough, I generally like to see my customers every six months. It is debatable if it is needed, but I like to do it. For some Patients, a six-month visit is an imperative, for others, twelve monthly visits would probably be fine.

The issue for us is that we don't know which is which until we have some experience with them. Undertaking six monthly appointments makes me feel comfortable that I am heading off any problems before they really happen. These ongoing callbacks will continue until the hearing aids die which will be for at least eight to ten years probably.

Occasional drop-in visits, Geoff they stopped working, you forgot to change your wax guards, oh yes sorry about that, how are the kids? Happens all the time, sometimes it isn't just wax guards.

Not justification, just information

I am not trying to justify prices here; I am simply trying to explain what goes into my assessment of price. I personally will probably spend at least twenty hours with a customer during the lifetime of an aid, I think my time and expertise is worth money. It is as simple as that.

I also have business expenses to cover, light heat, a receptionist, equipment costs rent and rates etc... These things all affect the price I set for hearing aids, is my retail price the same as others? Maybe, maybe not, however, I feel that the price I charge is commensurate with the level of care, attention and experience I provide.

The key here is that I have carefully made you aware of what I provide for the price I will charge. So you are very clear about what you are getting for the price I charge. What you need to understand is that what I offer may not be replicated by another provider. That is your job to both understand and assess.

Will a corporate business or another independent dispenser supply you with the same level of care and attention? Will their Dispenser have the same professional experience and expertise? If the answer is yes, well then you are assessing like for like.

There has been much talk about the greed of professionals, in particular in the United States. I can't comment on it because again, I don't know what the prices are or what the price includes. I also don't know what a professional considers a good hourly rate is over there.

If you are in the United States and looking for hearing aids, I think you can probably make a better assessment of that. The key learning I want to pass to you here is to understand what the price you pay includes, because if you understand that implicitly, you will be able to make an educated assessment of the benefit to cost ratio.

The last thing I will say is that just because it is cheaper, doesn't mean it is the same. Always understand the wider picture and be sure of exactly what you are getting for the prices you are paying. Always make sure you get it in writing.

Changing prices internationally

Hearing aid prices have been changing internationally over the last few years. There is a downward pressure on prices across the world that is mainly driven by low price sellers. In essence, many of these are internet based sellers that actually have no staff. What they do is generate leads that they pass onto private practices. The private practice is then forced to either sell the devices that you are interested in at the price dictated or they switch sell you to something else.

Many national businesses have also reduced their pricing based on the model that they are delivering. For instance, some in the UK and Ireland probably have some of the lowest pricing available. That pricing is realised through their business model, which in essence is a conveyor belt. Get them in, get them fitted, and see them when you can.

I don't agree with that business model, but hey, it works for them and there are plenty of people who buy from them. Do those people buy from them a second time? Of that, I am not sure, but I regularly have their customers come to me for help. I generally tell them to go back and demand help, which is what they paid for.

Experienced users of hearing aids tend not to base their buying decisions on price, although of course price is a factor. Experienced users are focused on service and care while new users with little experience focus solely on price. This fact and the pricing of others has led to reducing hearing aid prices overall.

A good thing and a bad thing

For the consumer, this has to be seen as a good thing right? Well yes and maybe no, but let me explain. There was definitely room to reduce prices; however, I think that providers also need to be careful. If we reduce our prices so much that it makes no financial sense. The consumer is the one that will suffer. I said it earlier, just because it walks like a duck, quacks like a duck, doesn't mean it is the same duck!

It is a simple equation if my price does not cover service, I either don't give it or I go out of business. It really is as simple as that. I think the death of Independent hearing healthcare providers would be a very bad thing for the consumer generally. Independents really do tend to act as checks and balances on the system. So, how can I address the downward pressure on prices but also make sure that the prices I charge make financial sense for my business and the consumers I serve?

Unbundled pricing

For many years there has been some debate within the profession about unbundling the pricing. By that, I mean clearly setting out the price of the hearing aid and the price portion of the service and care. While some, particularly in the states, have gone down that route it is by no means widespread. I think it is a great idea because it implicitly informs a consumer what they are buying.

It could also open up the pricing arrangements; for instance, say you didn't think that you would need any more than one check-up a year because you are a confident, experienced user. I think I would be willing to deduct the costs of the extra check-up and set a cost with you for any incidental appointments that arose.

There are some problems with using a system like this in the UK and Ireland because of the V.A.T. implications. It would mean hearing health providers who went down that route would have to begin to charge value-added tax for the services they implicitly provide. It is something that we would have to consider.

For me, I think that is a winner for both of us, you get a deduction and I am still covered for my time. I don't know how others in the industry feel about that and I am not sure how you feel about that, but I think it is something worth exploring. That is my personal opinion folks, for what it is worth, I don't know how others within the business feel.

In finishing, hearing aids are expensive, there is no getting away from that fact. However, you are buying far more than a simple electronic product.

Hearing Aid Manufacturers

The Hearing Aid Brands

There are many hearing aid brands across the world, in particular in the US. There is also a host of new players becoming involved globally. However, the hearing aid space is dominated by the big six. They are the biggest players in manufacturing globally and have the biggest market shares.

The big six is made up of Widex, Starkey, Signia (formerly Siemens), GN Resound, Sonova (who own Phonak and Unitron, and finally William Demant (who own Oticon and Bernafon). These manufacturers are the ones who dominate the global market and they do so for good reason. They offer some of the best hearing aids available today.

In the next few pages, I would like to try and give you a high-level overview of who they are and what they offer. I will not cover them all though, I will explain a few.

Widex

Renowned Danish Hearing Aid Brand

Widex is a Danish manufacturer who has been around since the fifties. They were founded by two men who had left William Demant and they first manufactured out of a garage. Since that beginning, Widex has become famous for technical excellence and an absolutely fantastic sound quality.

Widex has always followed its own agenda since its inception, their devices are firmly based in audiological research and because of it, and the strategies they use tend to be unique. For instance, they believe that the very soft sounds of speech are very important for understanding. So they amplify them to fit within your residual hearing.

This presents its own technical problems and Widex was one of the only manufacturers to do it up to recently. That is just one example of what they have done differently. Let's talk about the Widex range.

Widex Hearing Aids

Widex hearing aids have been renowned for their sound for as long as I remember. They are also famous for their high quality and reliability. In the recent past their hearing aids have been released on a platform which has four levels of technology and a family of hearing aid models. It appears that this is the way they will continue to launch hearing aids in the future, so it is worth me explaining.

The Platform

As I said, Widex changed the way they designated their hearing aids with the launch of the Clear platform in 2009. Since then, they have named their hearing aid platforms using one name such as Clear, Dream and just lately Unique. Within the platform are a full range of Widex hearing aid types and four levels of hearing aid technology.

Widex Unique Hearing Aids

Widex has a full line of hearing aids in every family normally, the new Beyond is different, but I will explain that a little later. So that means within the Unique platform, they offer Behind The Ear devices (BTE), Receiver in canal Devices (RIC) and custom In The Ear devices (ITE). Those devices would include:

CIC-M : This is the smallest of the range of custom ITE hearing aids; it is a non-wireless micro completely in canal device using a size 10 battery.

CIC: This is a slightly larger custom ITE device; it is a wireless completely-in-canal device using again a size 10 battery

Custom: This is a newly introduced wireless hearing aid model, it is in between the CIC and the XP but it offers a lot more versatility. For the first time in a long time, these devices will offer physical controls which mean you can have a volume control or a programme button on them. Unfortunately, the device will not have a telecoil. They are run on a 312 battery which means longer battery life.

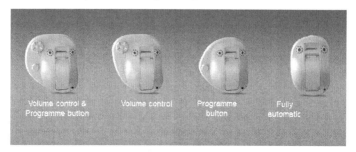

XP: The XP is for all intent and purposes a half shell type custom ITE device. It is a wireless in-the-ear device with a telecoil using a Size 312 battery

PASSION: The Passion has for many years been the smallest RIC hearing aid available but it has lost that honour to the new Unitron Now. It is a wireless mini receiver-in-canal device which uses a Size 10 battery. The size does limit the device though; it has no telecoil or programme button.

FUSION: The Fusion is a larger wireless receiver-in-canal device; it comes with a push button and telecoil and runs on a size 312 battery.

FASHION: The Fashion was introduced a couple of years ago as a replacement for the original 9 and 19 configurations, it is wireless slimline power BTE which can be used with a thin tube or a standard tube and mould. It has a volume control and telecoil and is powered by a size 312 battery.

Fashion Power: Pretty much exactly the same as the Fashion but designed to deliver for profound hearing losses.

FASHION Mini: The Fashion Mini was introduced in 2016 as a replacement for the original M configuration; it is wireless slimline mini BTE which can be used with a thin tube or a standard tube and mould. It is an exceptionally discreet BTE and is powered by a size 312 battery. It offers the discretion of a RIC with the reliability of a BTE, an excellent combination.

Each of these hearing aid types would be available in the four levels of technology available from Widex within that platform. For instance, there is a Widex Unique CIC-M 440, 330, 220 and 110 available. Let's talk about the technology levels.

The Widex Beyond

The Widex Beyond is a new addition; it is both a hearing aid type and platform. It is the very first Made For iPhone hearing aid from Widex. It is available only in a Fusion type device but it is available in the usual four technology levels. The Beyond offers a direct connection to an iPhone and comes with an accompanying app that gives you a lot of power over the function of your hearing aids. If you use an iPhone, the device is worth considering.

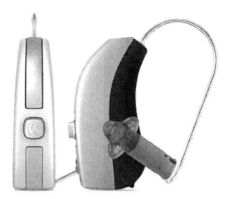

Widex have also introduced a rechargeable version of the Beyond which uses the rather excellent Z-Power silver-zinc rechargeable battery technology.

Widex technology levels

The premium level of technology in all of the recent Widex devices has been the 440. The technology levels drop via the 330, 220 and finally the 110. The technology levels are differentiated by features, the one with the latest and best Widex features is always the 440.

Technology levels are always something that confuses prospective buyers, in essence, each technology level offers the ability to hear clearly in different situations. The premium range offers the best support in every situation you will find yourself in. The entry level will offer much less support.

That isn't necessarily a bad thing; maybe you don't need the support! A good analogy is a Sat-Nav on a car; you can have a shiny new care with a pretty and sexy Sat-Nav. However, if you only go to the local shops, it is neither much use or worth paying for.

Hearing aid technologies are similar in concept, if you aren't very active socially, why would you want to pay for a level of technology that offers you the best support for hearing in complex sound situations? It is a lovely thing to have, but if you have no need for it, why bother or be worried about it?

I explain technology levels later in the book; however, I just think it is worthwhile making the comment here in our first introduction to manufacturers.

Phonak

Quality Swiss Technology

Phonak is a Swiss manufacturer of hearing aids who are owned by Sonova. They are one are one of the biggest hearing aid manufacturers in the world. They have been manufacturing hearing aids for over half a century and provide their devices in over 100 countries around the world. While they were once known for hearing aids for Children, they have become known for outstanding hearing aid technology that is suitable for all.

Phonak are rated as one of the best hearing aid manufacturers around today and they consistently work to improve their technology. Any experience I have had with Phonak hearing aids has been a good one and customers are consistently impressed with the benefit they provide.

Phonak Hearing Aids

Phonak do things a little differently than the other manufacturers when it comes to naming their hearing aids. They do introduce their hearing aids as platforms that are easily identifiable and they do use numbers to signify technology level. However, they split their hearing aid types with different names.

For instance, a flagship or premium range hearing aid from Phonak will use the number 90 while a basic aid will have the number 30 in the name. Their BTEs are called Bolero, their ITEs are called Virto and their RIC / RITEs are called Audeo. They also offer super power hearing aids named Naida.

The Platform

The Belong platform is now fully available and it is Phonak's latest hearing aid platform. Currently, the older Venture platform is still available. The Venture platform was a pretty good hearing aid range, so if you are offered it at a heavy discount, consider it. Just be aware that it is an older platform and ensure the price reflects it.

The Hearing Aids

All of the following hearing aids with the exception of the Audeo-BR, the Audeo B-Direct and the Bolero B-PR are available in four levels of technology.

Audeo Hearing Aids

With the Venture platform (older platform of Phonak hearing aids), there were four models of Audeo which were the V-10, which takes a size 10 battery, the Audeo V-312 which takes a size 312 battery. The Audeo V-312T which was the same again but with the addition of a telecoil receiver for a loop system and finally the Audeo V-13 which was the largest and fits a size 13 battery.

However, with the introduction of the Belong platform that has changed. The Audeo Belong range has five different types.

Audeo B-10: Very small RIC device using a size 10 battery, it is quite discreet and can be used with several receiver variations meaning it can cover a lot of hearing losses. It doesn't have a telecoil although as always it is a wireless device. It has a button but no volume control.

Audeo B-312: Again a very small RIC device, however, it uses a size 312 battery, it is still very discreet and can be used with several receiver variations meaning it can cover a lot of hearing losses. Like the 10, it doesn't have a telecoil although as always it is a wireless device. It has a button but no volume control.

Audeo B-312T: Slightly bigger than the 312, it is still a small and discrete device RIC which uses a size 312 battery; it can be used with several receiver variations meaning it can cover a lot of hearing losses. Unlike the 10 and the 312, it has a telecoil as well as being a wireless device. It has a button but no volume control.

Audeo B-13: The largest of the Audeo B RIC range, it runs on a size 13 battery and can be used with several receiver variations meaning it can cover a lot of hearing losses. The 13 comes fully loaded with a telecoil, programme button and a volume control as well as being a wireless device.

Audeo B-R: The RIC device that all the hype of late has been about, a rechargeable hearing device running on Lithium-ion power. A solid 24 hours of use from one three hour charge. It can be used with several receiver variations meaning it can cover a lot of hearing losses down to profound. It is also a wireless device with a programme button but no volume control or telecoil. The Audeo B-R is only available in the top three levels of technology though and not the entry level.

Audeo B-Direct

A new addition to the Audeo range is the Audeo B-Direct hearing aids which Phonak are billing as Made For Any Phone. These are really very interesting devices that offer a direct connection to any Bluetooth enabled mobile phone. They are a first and a unique offering.

It is really a revolutionary hearing aid that changes wireless connection to a mobile phone forever. The Audeo B-Direct connects to any Bluetooth® enabled mobile phone, directly without a streamer. Even better, it offers true hands-free calling. As it supports the classic Bluetooth protocol, it provides direct connectivity to cell phones – including Android, iPhone® and even classic cell phones – with no extra body-worn streaming device required.

True hands-free calling is now a reality

The hearing aids offer real hands-free voice calling. The wearer can answer or reject a phone call by simply pressing the push button on their hearing aid. The ringing of the phone is heard through the hearing aids and once the call is accepted, the conversation is instantly streamed. You don't even need to pick up your phone. Your voice is picked up by the hearing aid's intelligent microphone network and transmitted to the other caller similar to a wireless headset.

No Music Streaming

Unfortunately for people who like to stream music or audio books from their phone, this hearing device isn't the answer. While it delivers astonishing new power over mobile phone calls, it doesn't allow the type of streaming that delivers music or other audio. However, they have thought about music lovers and your TV viewing habits.

Hearing aids that double as wireless TV headphones

They have also introduced an accompanying TV Connector, which uses their proprietary AirStreamTM technology. It is designed to be a state-of-the-art compact multimedia hub that seamlessly connects wearers to their favourite TV programming for an immersive audio experience. It's a plug and play solution that automatically turns a pair of Audéo B-Direct hearing aids into wireless TV headphones. The TV Connector can also connect and transmit to multiple sets of Audéo B-Direct hearing aids simultaneously.

Three levels of technology

The new device will be available in three levels of technology, the 90, the 70 and the 50, so no entry level device this time around. Although that was to be expected based on the introduction of the rechargeable devices.

New Accompanying App

There is a new app to go with the devices for smartphones; the app offers the typical features you would expect.

Volume adjustment, programme changes, you can also rename the programmes to make them easier to remember. The app will show a list of the available audio sources and allow the user to control the balance of audio when streaming.

Virto Hearing Aids

The full Virto Belong hearing aid range has now been delivered and it includes the new Titanium model. Phonak say that the Virto B is the world's first hearing aids with Biometric Calibration, which take your individual ear anatomy and hearing needs into account.

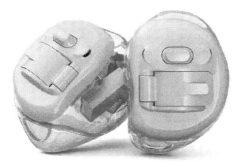

They say that they will identify over 1600 biometric data points in and on your ear, and the unique calibration settings are calculated for each Virto B hearing aid. In this way,

Virto B is able to more reliably sense where the sound is coming from, thereby giving you access to a better hearing performance.

Using The Outer Ear

Phonak are the first ever hearing aid manufacturer to carefully map the outer ear to take advantage of its natural abilities. The outer ear naturally heightens some sounds while also helping us to identify where sounds are coming from. They say that this new process will deliver a 2dB signal to noise ratio improvement. Basically means it will make the signal (what you want to listen to) 2dB higher than the noise. 2dB doesn't sound like much but combined with all the other strategies that Phonak use it will be a marked improvement.

Fully Automatic

The Virto hearing aids are fully automatic and run on their latest AutoSense OS™. The Virto B is available in six models to match your hearing needs.

Four Levels of Technology

It is also available in the usual four levels of technology, the 90, 70, 50 and 30. They say that there will also be a Virto B CROS.

The currently available Virto hearing aids are:

Virto B-10 NW O: This is the smallest of the devices. The 10 means it takes a size 10 battery, NW means no wireless so you miss out on all of the features for which wireless is needed. O stands for omnidirectional which means that you don't get the benefits associated with dual microphones.

Virto B-10 O: This is the same as the previous model but with wireless technology.

Virto B-10: This is again the same as the others but with dual microphones squeezed on.

Virto B-312 NW O: This device is actually a slightly larger mini-canal device with a 312 battery, unfortunately, to get the discretion, you lose out on the wireless features and you only get omnidirectional microphones.

Virto B-312: This device is a larger "half shell" aid that takes a size 312 battery.

Virto B-13: This is a "full shell" aid that takes a size 13 battery.

Virto B-Titanium Invisible Hearing Aids

This device is quite ground-breaking; it is the first hearing aid device to use medical grade titanium to form the custom shell. While this alone is innovative, they have used the properties of the metal to ensure that they can offer discreet custom hearing aids to more people than ever.

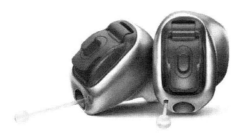

A Titanium Shell

Phonak named the hearing aid as the Virto B-Titanium and said it will be the most discreet in-ear device they have ever made. It is a fascinating device that uses titanium for the shell instead of the usual hard acrylic. This is the first time that titanium has been used in the manufacture of a custom hearing aid.

Super discreet

Virto B-Titanium is the smallest Phonak in-the-ear hearing aid ever! It is for all intent and purpose an invisible hearing aid device.

Half as Thin

Using titanium allows for a shell that's half as thin as traditional custom shells. This will result in a deep, comfortable fit. Phonak say that the overall size is reduced significantly, thus increasing invisible-in-the-canal (IIC) fit rate by 64%. That simply means that more people than ever will be physically suitable for their latest invisible hearing aid.

Three Levels of Receiver

The device comes available with three levels of receiver which allows it to cover even more hearing losses than ever before. Because of the use of Titanium, it also allows for bigger vents in their hearing aids which mean fewer occlusion problems for people with good low-frequency hearing.

Fully automatic

Virto B-Titanium features AutoSense OS™. It adapts to every sound environment automatically for excellent hearing performance everywhere. There will be no need to manually adjust the hearing aids. Although, they can come with an optional push button for just that.

Technology Levels

The Virto B-Titanium will only be available in the 90 and the 70 levels of technology.

Will Fit More People Than Ever

The material is exceptionally strong, which allows Phonak to make the shell much thinner than ever before with even more strength. This combined with new component design allows them to deliver an invisible hearing device that they say will fit 68% more ears.

Bolero Belong Hearing Aids

With the launch of the new Bolero Belong platform of BTE hearing aids, Phonak have launched the anticipated lithium-ion rechargeable BTE, the Bolero B-PR. It is the first Lithium-ion rechargeable BTE to the market and the first rechargeable BTE for Phonak. They say that the battery pack will deliver 24 hours of hearing with one simple charge (expected results when fully charged, and up to 80 minutes wireless streaming time) which is in line with the performance of the Audeo B-R.

The P hearing aid style is quite a powerful aid and can be expected to be fitted to people with severe hearing loss. The device has a programme button, volume control and a telecoil on board. The amplification output of this aid demands a lot of power, so Phonak must be very confident with the battery technology.

In line with the Audeo Belong, the range will run on the new improved AutoSense OS and will come in the usual four levels of technology. However, the new rechargeable option will not be available in the lowest level of technology.

The Range

The Bolero range is a full model line up with four models. They will include B-M, B-P, B-SP, and the rechargeable B-PR.

Phonak Bolero B-M: The B-M model is the smallest of the range, a micro BTE powered with a 312 battery it will cover Moderate to Severe hearing losses. The device comes with a programme button and has an onboard telecoil. The device can be fitted with a thin tube fitting or a traditional tube and mould configuration. The device will be available in the four levels of technology, the 90, the 70, the 50 and the 30.

Phonak Bolero B-P: The B-P model is slightly larger, it is powered by a 13 battery cell and comes with a programme button, volume control, telecoil and will cover up to severe hearing losses. The device can be fitted with a thin tube fitting or a traditional tube and mould configuration. The device will be available in the four levels of technology, the 90, the 70, the 50 and the 30.

Bolero B-SP: The B-SP is the largest model; again it is powered by a 13 battery and comes with a programme button, volume control and telecoil. The device will cover severe to profound hearing losses. The device can be fitted with a thin tube fitting or a traditional tube and mould configuration. The device will be available in the four levels of technology, the 90, the 70, the 50 and the 30.

Bolero B-PR: The B-PR is the rechargeable model which runs on a sealed and integrated lithium-ion power pack. The device is similar in size to the Bolero B-SP. It also has a programme button, volume control and telecoil. The device can be fitted with a thin tube fitting or a traditional tube and mould configuration. It will cover moderate to severe hearing losses and it will be available in the 90, the 70 and the 50 levels of technology only.

Naida Hearing Aids

Again the Naida is currently only available on the Venture platform. It was the last of the Venture platform to be released and I would not expect it to be updated for a while. The currently available Naida hearing aids are:

Naida V RIC: The Naida V RIC (Receiver in Canal) offers pretty amazing power in a small package. The device which is a new form factor with a size 13 battery comes with three possible receiver options, the XS, the XP and the new X UP (for Ultra Power). The X UP option is a newly designed receiver which offers more output than the previous one. In essence, the option will cover a more severe hearing loss.

Naida V SP: The new Naida V SP is quite a small superpower hearing aid. It runs on a size thirteen battery and can be fitted with a power slim tube and tip which offers real discretion. The device can also be fitted with a standard thick tube and mould configuration. The SP runs on a size thirteen battery which accounts for that smaller size.

Naida V UP: The new Naida V UP is again thinner and smaller than its predecessor with a new form factor. The power output of the hearing aid has been increased giving it, even more, performance for even the most profound hearing loss. It is powered by a 675 battery and can also be fitted with a power slim tube and custom tip.

Phonak Hearing Aid Technology

Phonak hearing aid technology comes in four levels of technology that are numbered, the 90 is the top of the range and it drops through the 70, the 50 and finally the 30 which is the bottom of the range.

Starkey

American Hearing Aids

Starkey is an American hearing aid manufacturer who became famous for their custom hearing aids. They produced very discreet custom hearing aids at a time that others had problems doing it. They are exceptionally popular in the States and there are more than a few providers in the UK that use them as a primary manufacturer. I don't like them, their hearing aid technology has always seemed okay, but I had a lot of problems with reliability. So much so that I just stopped using them.

At the time of going to press, Starkey were making a raft of announcements at their major yearly event in Las Vegas. One of the announcements was about a brand new type of rechargeable hearing aid which would be run with a Lithium-Ion battery pack.

The other was slightly cryptic about a hearing aid to be released this year which would have onboard sensors which could track movement, detect falls, track activity and instantly translate languages.

I for one have hoped to see something like this for many years and I am looking forward to seeing the devices when they are released. Keep an eye on Hearing Aid Know for the details when they are released.

Starkey Hearing Aids

Starkey is similar to the other manufacturers when it comes to naming their hearing aids. They do introduce their hearing aids as platforms that are easily identifiable and they do use numbers to signify technology level. However, they too divide different hearing aid types with different names.

For instance, a flagship or premium range hearing aid from Starkey will use the number i2400 while a basic aid will have the number i1600 in the name. Their full line hearing aid offering is called Muse IQ, their IIC hearing aids are called SoundLens Synergy IQ and their Made For iPhone hearing aids are called Halo IQ.

The Platform

Starkey has a few hearing aid platforms floating around right now; the latest is called the IQ platform. All of the hearing aid types I will discuss use that platform.

SoundLens Synergy IQ

The SoundLens was the first of the modern invisible hearing aids. While they are not suitable for everyone, they seem to be pretty solid devices. Anyone I have ever come across wearing them has been very impressed with them. The Starkey SoundLens Synergy IQ comes in two styles:

Starkey SoundLens Wireless: This is a wireless (invisible-in-canal) device; however, it is only available in the premium range i2400.

Starkey SoundLens Non-Wireless: This is a non-wireless (invisible-in-canal) hearing aid and it is available at all tech levels.

Muse IQ

The Muse IQ range comes in a variety of styles:

Starkey Muse Mini BTE: This is a wireless BTE device, powerful but discreet traditional type BTE hearing aid. With rocker switch and telecoil (size 312 battery).

Starkey Muse BTE 13: This is a wireless BTE device, powerful but discreet traditional type BTE hearing aid. With rocker switch and telecoil (size 13 battery).

Starkey Muse Micro RIC 312t: This is a wireless mini RIC (receiver-in-canal) device, small, ultra-discreet but powerful hearing solution. With push button and multiflex tinnitus therapy (size 312 battery).

Starkey Muse RIC 312t: This is a wireless RIC (receiver-in-canal) device, larger than the micro RIC but still a discreet but powerful hearing solution. With push button and multiflex tinnitus therapy (size 312 battery).

Starkey Muse CIC: This is a wireless CIC (completely-in-canal) device, small, ultra-discreet but powerful hearing solution with optional telecoil depending on the size of the canal (Size 10/312 battery).

Starkey Muse ITC: This is a wireless ITC (in-the-canal) device, small, ultra-discreet but powerful hearing solution, with a telecoil (Size 312 battery).

Starkey Muse ITE: This is a wireless ITE (in-the-ear) device, a powerful custom hearing solution with a telecoil (Size 13 battery).

The Halo IQ

Starkey was the second manufacturer to introduce Made For iPhone hearing aids and this is their third update of them. I have personally worn the Halo 2 devices at the premium range and I have to say they were pretty good devices. Nice crisp sound, good connection to the iPhone and great power delivered through the app. The Halo IQ range is a Made For iPhone technology which comes in four styles all of which are receiver in canal devices:

Starkey Halo IQ RIC 312: This is a wireless RIC (receiver-in-canal) device, small, ultra-discreet but powerful hearing solution. With push button and multiflex tinnitus therapy (size 13 battery).

Starkey Halo IQ RIC 13: This is a wireless RIC (receiver-in-canal) device, small, ultra-discreet but powerful hearing solution. With push button and multiflex tinnitus therapy (size 13 battery).

Starkey Halo IQ RIC 312 AP: This is a wireless RIC (receiver-in-canal) device, small, ultra-discreet but powerful hearing solution. With push button and multiflex tinnitus therapy (size 13 battery). This device will cover very severe hearing losses.

Starkey Halo IQ RIC 13 AP: This is a wireless RIC (receiver-in-canal) device, small, ultra-discreet but powerful hearing solution. With push button and multiflex tinnitus therapy (size 13 battery). This device will cover very severe hearing losses.

Starkey Technology Levels

Starkey keeps to three levels of technology in its latest platform, the Premium i2400, the Advanced i2000, the Standard i1600. All of the hearing aids we have discussed here are available in those three levels.

Signia

Signia /Sivantos /Siemens

Siemens is a well-known German company and their hearing aid division was one of the largest manufacturers of hearing aids worldwide. They sold their hearing aid division to a private consortium named Sivantos a couple of years ago. Sivantos have now changed the hearing aid brand to Signia but they are still dual branded with Siemens. This is something that will slowly change over the next couple of years.

I think that Signia bear watching over the next few years, I think if anyone will break the mould it will be them. While there technology is based on real pedigree and decades of research, the company itself has no baggage and no real history within the business.

I think this frees them from a lot of the thought processes that govern other hearing aid brands. If I were to bet on a manufacturer to be first into the Over The Counter market, I would bet on Signia. Probably lose my shirt though.

Signia Hearing Aids

Up to now, Signia has been similar to Phonak when it comes to naming their hearing aids. They do introduce their hearing aids as platforms that are easily identifiable and they do use numbers to signify technology level. However, they split their hearing aid types with different names.

For instance, a flagship or premium range hearing aid from Signia will use the number 7 while a basic aid will have the number 3 in the name. Their BTEs are called Motion, their ITEs are called Insio and their RIC / RITEs up to now have been called Ace, Pure, carat and Cellion. They also offer super power hearing aids named Nitro.

They offer a whole range of other cheaper platforms that I am not going to cover here as well.

Telecare 3.0

This is a really interesting development; Signia has made the Telecare service a live service. They were initially the first to offer Telecare with a limited fine-tuning option although Resound quickly followed with the launch of the LiNX 3D and their Remote Assist which had more functionality. Signia though quickly expanded that fine-tuning option and added video calling to the system. Now they have enabled full live remote tuning with video support which is a pretty huge breakthrough.

The new service means that you can set-up a video call with your hearing professional and explain the issue you are having in the situation you are having it in. While you are connected, your hearing professional can tweak your hearing aid's settings live and you can quickly assess if they are better.

The Platform

Signia have two platforms right now that can be called the latest, they have just introduced their Nx platform or at least some of the hearing aids from that platform. The currently also have the Primax platform available which was actually an outstanding set of hearing aids. I am going to detail what is available on the Nx at present and I will also discuss the Primax offerings.

Signia Nx Hearing Aids

Signia introduced the Nx hearing aids late in 2017, it is a completely new platform and it comes with some outstanding new features.

Made For iPhone

The entire Nx range is Made For iPhone enabled hearing aids that offer a direct connection to Apple devices for audio streaming.

OVP, Own Voice Processing

Signia made a big deal of the OVP or Own Voice Processing at the launch, and these devices are the first hearing aids to process the user's own voice differently from everything else. In fact, they have dedicated a completely separate processor on the platform to facilitate that. They said that the strategy will increase the acceptance of a user's own voice dramatically.

I Second That

I have to agree wholeheartedly with that sentiment, the OVP feature is amazing. My experience with it has been pretty jaw-dropping. In the article **Signia Pure 312 7 Nx Hearing Aids, Here is What You Need to Know**, I talked in more depth about the own voice processing feature and why it might be of interest to you. The pertinent statement here though is:

When I was fitted with the Nx I was fitted with closed domes, I thought this isn't going to work as I heard my voice explode in my head. Then, we went through the own voice training protocol (count from twenty-one until it is happy it knows your voice). The feature was turned on, and no more occlusion, just like that. I was a bit speechless (that doesn't happen very often). By no more occlusion I mean no more auditory occlusion, I wasn't caused any difficulty by my own voice.

For new users of hearing aids the sound quality of their own voice can be off-putting, but it is usually something that they get used to. However, as Signia point out, used to, does not mean happy with. This system promises to deal with the issue and it does it exceptionally well.

Three Models, Three Levels of Tech

There are three models initially available across three levels of technology. As is the norm with Signia tech levels naming system, the levels are the premium 7, the mid-range 5 and the entry level 3. The models themselves are two Receiver In Canal devices and a BTE.

Pure 13 NX

This device is an updated version of their Pure 13 BT, it offers the new system which separately processes the wearer's own voice. It comes with superior connectivity with direct streaming and the myControl App which deliver personal control over the devices. The hearing aid has a rocker switch which allows programme changes and volume changes. It is IP68 rated and can be fitted with the four levels of receiver power making it suitable for most hearing losses. Signia say that users will enjoy the longest wearing time in its class while streaming. It also has access to the full live remote support via TeleCare 3.0.

Pure 312 Nx

This device is a very svelte Pure (RIC) device using a 312 battery, again it offers the new system which separately processes the wearer's own voice. The hearing aid has a rocker switch which allows programme changes and volume changes. It is IP68 rated. It can also be fitted with the four levels of receiver making it suitable for most hearing losses.

It comes with superior connectivity with direct streaming and the myControl App. It also has access to the full live remote support via TeleCare 3.0.

Motion 13 Nx

This device is a BTE device using a 13 battery, again it offers the new system which separately processes the wearer's own voice. It also comes with superior connectivity with direct streaming and the myControl App. It also has access to the full live remote support via TeleCare 3.0. The device also offers the rocker switch for programme and volume control changes. This is a pretty versatile device which offers a telecoil option with the simple switching of the battery door. The device is IP67 rated for dust and moisture.

Primax Hearing Aids

All of the following hearing aids are available in three levels of technology.

RIC Hearing Aids

Signia offers three receiver in canal hearing aids in the Primax range, the Ace, the Pure and the Cellion:

Signia Ace Primax: This is a light and comfortable solution, Ace Primax is the smallest in their family of RIC hearing aids. It is an ideal solution for first-time users offering both discretion and functionality. It can deliver real power and comes in a tiny form.

Pure Primax Hearing Aids: This solution offers more control over the hearing aids. The new Pure Primax combines elegant looks with the power of Primax technology in a RIC hearing aid. The devices are suitable for almost every hearing loss. They are also available in the older rechargeable option from Signia.

Cellion Primax hearing aids: Outstanding rechargeable hearing aid with lithium-ion charging. Ideal for any user who doesn't want the hassle of changing batteries. It's rechargeable lithium-ion power cell lasts up to two days without charging, while it's unique design makes it hassle-free and easy to use.

Signia Behind The Ear Hearing Aids

Signia offers four Behind The Ear hearing aids in the Motion range the Motion Sx, the Motion SA, the Motion S and the Motion P which is the most powerful:

Motion Primax SX: The Motion SX is a wireless rechargeable BTE that can be fitted with a thin-tube or standard BTE tubing and mould. It has a volume control, telecoil and uses a size 13 battery.

Motion Primax SA: The Motion SA is a wireless BTE that can be fitted with a thin-tube or standard BTE tubing and mould. It has a volume control, telecoil and uses a size 13 battery.

Motion Primax PX: The Motion PX is a wireless high-power rechargeable BTE that can be used with a thin-tube or standard BTE tubing and mould. It has a push button, volume control and telecoil. It also uses a size 13 battery.

Signia In The Ear Hearing Aids

Signia offers four In The Ear hearing aids in the Insio range, the Insio IIC, the Insio CIC, the Insio ITC and the Insio ITE:

Insio Primax IIC: The IIC is a non-wireless invisible-in-canal hearing aid that uses a size 10 battery.

Insio Primax CIC: The Insio CIC is a wireless completely-in-canal device that uses a size 10 battery.

Insio Primax ITC: The Insio ITC is a wireless in-the-canal hearing aid with telecoil and it can be ordered with a size 10 or 312 battery.

Insio Primax ITE: The Insio ITE is a wireless full shell in-the-ear hearing aid with telecoil and it can be ordered with a size 312 or 13 battery.

Signia Technology Levels

As I said there are three levels of technology, the Premium 7px, the Advanced 5px, the Standard 3px. All of the hearing aids we have discussed here are available in those three levels.

GN Resound

Danish Manufacturer Famous for Made For iPhone

GN Resound is another Danish hearing aid manufacturer with a long history. They are one of the top 5 manufacturers in the world and are renowned for innovation and constantly advancing technology. Since they began in the 1940's, Resound has continued to grow but it is in the last 20 years their innovation has pushed them to new heights.

They have had a lot of firsts over the years; their latest first was Made For iPhone hearing aids. They are still the only manufacturer that offers a full range of Made For iPhone (MFI) hearing aids including BTEs, RICs and ITEs.

Resound Hearing Aids

Resound are similar to the other manufacturers when it comes to naming their hearing aids. They introduce their hearing aids as platforms that are easily identifiable and they do use numbers to signify technology level. Each platform would have a full range of hearing aids available

For instance, a flagship or premium range hearing aid from Resound will use the number 9 while a basic aid will have the number 5 in the name. Their latest hearing aid offering is called the LiNX 3D.

The Platform

Resound have a few hearing aid platforms floating around right now, the very latest is called the Linx 3D platform. However, they also have the Enzo 3D range which is an MFI (Made For iPhone) superpower hearing aid range for people with profound hearing loss and the Verso which is a non MFI, wireless hearing aid range and the Vea, which again is a budget non MFI, wireless hearing aid range.

Linx 3D Hearing Aids

The LiNX 3D hearing aid range comes in a variety of styles that include:

IIC Invisible in Canal: This is a non-wireless invisible-in-canal device. It uses a size 10 battery. So it really isn't a Made For iPhone device.

CIC Completely in Canal: This is again a non-wireless completely-in-canal hearing aid. It uses a size 10 battery. Same as above when it comes to connectivity.

ITC In The Canal: This is a slightly larger wireless Made for iPhone in-the-canal hearing aid. It uses a size 312 battery.

ITE In The Ear: This is a larger full shell wireless Made for iPhone in-the-ear hearing with a telecoil. It uses a size 312 or 13 battery.

MIH-S Microphone in Helix Small: Resound are the only manufacturers who offer this style of hearing aid, it is a non-wireless small microphone-in-helix hearing device. The microphone is attached to a wire that is placed in the helix of your ear. It uses a size 10 battery.

MIH Microphone in Helix: This is a larger version of the wireless Made for iPhone microphone-in-helix hearing aid. This version has a telecoil. It uses a size 312 or 13 battery.

RIE 61: This is a wireless Made for iPhone receiver-in-ear hearing aid with a push button. It uses a size 312 battery.

RIE 62: This is a slightly larger wireless Made for iPhone receiver-in-ear hearing aid that is equipped with a volume control and telecoil. It uses a size 13 battery.

BTE 77: This is a wireless Made for iPhone BTE that can be used with a thin-tube or standard BTE tubing and mould. This device has a push button, volume control and telecoil. It uses a size 13 battery.

BTE 88: This is a wireless high-power Made for iPhone BTE. The device is fitted with a push button, volume control and telecoil. It uses a size 13 battery.

Enzo 3D Hearing Aids

The Enzo 3D superpower range is offered in two styles:

Enzo 3D 88 BTE: This is a wireless high-power Made for iPhone BTE. The device is fitted with a push button, volume control and telecoil. It uses a size 13 battery.

Enzo 3D 98 BTE: This is a wireless high-power Made for iPhone BTE. The device is fitted with a push button, volume control and telecoil. It uses a size 675 battery.

Resound Technology Levels

As I said there are three levels of technology in every Resound platform, in the ordinary ranges the levels are the Premium 9, the Advanced 7, and the Standard 5. With the introduction of the budget Vea range they did something different, they offered a 1, 2 and 3.

They also limited the types of hearing aids available in the range, for instance, there was no MIH in the Vea range. The range seems to have become obsolete and Resound seems to have removed it from their websites.

Hearing Aid Types

Hearing Aid Types, an introduction

Modern hearing aids have evolved exponentially in the last five years; they really are outstanding at what they do. One thing we will say though is that they are just an aid to hearing; they will not replace the natural hearing ability that you have lost.

That warning should not put you off, it is just given so that you can manage your expectations. It is also given so that you can appreciate what you are going to get. Our best advice is that you should buy the best set of hearing aids you can afford. The key is that you buy them from someone who is going to do their level best to help you succeed with them.

Best Advice

Because, if you have a hearing loss, you need to treat it. The growing evidence in relation to the consequences of untreated hearing loss is worrying. We are seeing stronger links between untreated hearing loss and cognitive issues. We are also seeing solid evidence that hearing aids have a beneficial effect on cognitive ability.

We as a population are generally living longer, it appears that treating hearing loss will keep you sharper, more active and generally healthier as you age. There is clear evidence that shows that wearing hearing aids when needed will contribute to good general health, so what's not to like?

Be realistic with your expectations of the hearing aids that you purchase, the different levels of technology make a big difference to the benefit delivered within different sound environments. We will explain them clearly a little later in the book.

While there is a vast range of hearing aids available they normally fall within just a few overall general types. Each type has different strengths and weaknesses and differing suitability for different people. Let's explore the different types including the pros and cons of each one.

What Are The Hearing Aid Types?

There are three hearing aid types that are most spoken about, they are as follows:

BTE Hearing Aids: These devices are worn with the hearing aid on top of and behind the ear. All of the parts are in the case at the back of the ear and they are joined to the ear canal with a sound tube and a custom mould or tip.

ITE Hearing Aids: These are custom-made devices, all of the electronics sit in a device that fits in your ear, and they come in many sizes including CIC (Completely in Canal) and IIC (Invisible in Canal).

RIC RITE Hearing Aids: These devices are similar in concept to BTE hearing aids, with the exception that the receiver (the speaker) has been removed from the case that sits at the back of the ear. It is fitted in your ear canal or ear and connected to the case of the hearing aid with a thin wire.

Bluetooth Hearing Aids, Wireless versus Non-Wireless Hearing Aids

Before we delve a little deeper into the different types of hearing aids it is important to discuss a new type that has become commonly known to the general public as Bluetooth hearing aids, but to us in the profession as wireless hearing aids. All of the hearing device manufacturers have introduced wireless hearing aids over the last few years.

Some have even introduced Made For iPhone hearing aids which we will discuss later. While some of them work with Bluetooth connections, they aren't exactly Bluetooth. However, just recently most of the hearing aid manufacturers have signed up to the single Bluetooth protocol so a standardised method is coming.

Most of the manufacturers have designed their own flavour of wireless signal. Wireless communication between hearing aids and between hearing aids and other accessory devices has really been a game changer for people who wear hearing aids.

Not just has it made it easier for people to enjoy their TV, phone calls and group situations, the wireless communication has also enabled jaw-dropping features (at least for us nerds) in the hearing aids that deliver a much better experience for their users.

As you can probably tell, I like wireless hearing aids. Some people choose discretion over wireless communications when choosing custom hearing aids. Honestly, and that is what this book is about, honesty, I think they are quite mad. Perhaps, certifiable. So in finishing, go wireless and you will never go back.

Receiver in Canal Hearing Aids

RIC Receiver in Canal Hearing Aids
RIC/ RITE hearing aids, sometimes called speaker in the ear, are powerful but discreet hearing aids. Let's take a deeper look at them.

The Most Popular Hearing Aids

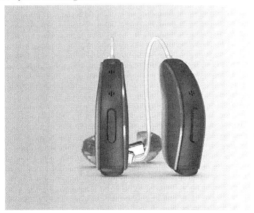

RIC (Receiver in Canal) / RITE (Receiver In The Ear) are relatively recent additions to the hearing aid world introduced around 2008 as far as I can remember. In an effort to produce ever smaller but more powerful Behind The Ear type hearing aids, manufacturers moved the receiver (the speaker part) out of the body of the hearing aid and placed it at the end of a wire that went into the ear canal. Hence, receiver in canal or receiver in the ear.

The devices have become hugely popular both within the profession and with buyers because they are massively versatile fitting many types of hearing losses and very discreet. In some cases, they are more discreet than in the ear hearing aids. They do however have their pros and cons, let's take a deeper look at them.

The Pros & Cons of RIC Hearing Aids

As with many things in life, there are pros and cons with RIC hearing aids, let's take a deeper look at those. First, let's take a look at the advantages of RIC devices.

What Are The Advantages Of RIC Devices?

Discreet

They are highly discreet devices; although the body of the hearing aid sits behind the ear they are normally very small and discreet. Unless someone is actually checking they invariably go unnoticed.

The wire that leads from the body of the hearing aid into the ear canal is tiny and should sit along the crease of your face at the ear, hence, it is almost unnoticeable as well. Because of these two facts, these are among the most discreet hearing aids available.

Easy Change Receivers

Because the receiver is easily interchangeable these hearing aids can cover varied hearing losses from mild all the way through to severe to profound. It also means that if the receiver fails, which happens, it is easily changed out for a new one.

This means that the hearing aid does not have to go away for repair for a receiver change, it can be done instantly in the office if the hearing professional has spare receivers. This is a big plus, being without your hearing aid once you are used to wearing it is excruciating.

The simple joy of being able to hear well without huge levels of concentration and straining is only something you appreciate after you have a problem with your hearing.

What Are the Disadvantages of RIC Devices

Receiver Issues in RICs/RITEs

The fact that the receiver is placed in the canal or the ear is both a blessing and curse. This placement exposes it to the hostile environment that the ear is for electronics. Your ear canal is wet warm and oily, all of the things that electronics tend not to like.

The manufacturers take great pains to protect the receivers with Nano coating materials, enclosed casings and wax guard protectors. However, unless you take good care of the receivers, changing your wax guards when you should, (you probably won't) inevitably wax gets into them.

At best, this can just block the sound outlet, at worst, it can ingress into the receiver itself and destroy it. Wax and moisture is the kiss of death for receivers. Thankfully, the receivers are easily replaced by your hearing professional; however, after the manufacturer's warranty is up you may have to pay for them.

While they vary in cost, they are not expensive, however, if you are replacing them regularly, the cost adds up. I don't want to put you off this device types, they are exceptionally versatile and I really like them. If you are recommended this type of device just be aware of the receiver issues.

Many of the hearing healthcare professionals we partner with can arrange a five-year manufacturer's warranty to cover repairs. Some may charge, some may actually offer it for free.

If you are considering buying RICs, ask about an extended manufacturer's warranty.

Maybe Too Small!

As I said, RICs / RITEs are very small and discreet devices, normally the smaller they are, the smaller the battery they use. Both the size of the hearing aid and the size of the battery can cause difficulties for people with dexterity issues. The whole idea of acquiring hearing aids is so that you can wear them and enjoy the very real benefits of hearing better.

If you have difficulty handling them to put them in, what should be a joy, can easily turn into a frustrating task at best.

The same has to be said about the batteries, small batteries can be a nightmare for people with vision or dexterity issues. Many of the hearing aid manufacturers offer RIC / RITE hearing aids in a variety of sizes and battery sizes, for instance, Phonak offer the

Audeo V range in a size 10 battery, a size 312 battery and a size 13 battery. The only caveat is the bigger the battery, the bigger the hearing aid case.

Contra-indications To Wearing RICs / RITEs

There are some people who shouldn't wear these type of devices. If you have permanent perforations in your ears or you have had a mastoid operation these hearing devices aren't really for you.

As you will know if you have these problems there is an increased risk of middle ear infections and fluid release. Either will destroy the receivers of the hearing aids, because of the nature of your ears with these conditions receiver failures would be an ongoing problem rather than an occasional frustration. The same can be said for people who suffer from wet ears or produce a large amount of earwax, either condition will cause issues for the receivers.

In Finishing

Great devices, pros and cons, good care will lead to fewer problems.

In The Ear Hearing Aids

ITE In The Ear Hearing Aids

In The Ear or custom hearing aids are discreet and popular hearing aids for consumers, let's take a deeper look at them.

Custom Hearing Aids

ITE, CIC, IIC HEARING AIDS

Custom hearing aids or in the ear hearing aids come in many shapes and sizes, from quite visible Full Shell hearing aids to the so-called hidden hearing aids, the Invisible In Canal or IICs.

Custom hearing aids have been around for a very long time, as I said they come in many shapes and sizes that deliver different levels of power and functionality. They were hugely popular devices but when RIC / RITE devices were introduced their popularity waned somewhat.

With the introduction of the so-called "Invisible hearing aids" several years ago there has been a resurgence in their popularity. Hearing aid manufacturers are also overcoming some of the technical challenges that reduced the functionality of the very small custom device types in the recent past.

This has made the devices a better choice for people who need more help in tougher environments but want a very discreet package. Many of the manufacturers now offer small completely in canal devices that are wireless enabled which eliminates the traditional trade-off between discretion and functionality. Let's talk about the types.

Invisible Hearing Aids

Invisible hearing aids or hidden hearing aids have been with us for a while, however, initially, they actually weren't that hidden. That has changed though over the last five years. The manufacturers cracked the difficulties that precluded them from making really invisible hearing aids.

Since then every manufacturer has introduced a truly invisible in the canal hearing aid range. They fit deeply in the ear canal and the faceplate cannot be seen easily. They are truly discreet hearing devices and they have been well received. There are of course disadvantages, the IIC hearing aids are often too small to be wireless.

However, in the recent past, some of the manufacturers, Starkey, Siemens and Oticon in particular, have delivered wireless IIC devices.

For some, the trade-off between discretion and wireless functionality is an easy choice. They forgo wireless capability for the discretion, however, I believe there is a lot to be said for wireless capability. I think wireless accessories are outstanding solutions and used well they have changed the lives of hard of hearing people dramatically for the better.

But hey, that's just me. Invisible hearing aids are not suitable for everyone for several reasons, some reasons I will discuss later when talking about the overall pros and cons of custom hearing aids. However, there is one that is particular to invisible hearing aids, canal size and shape. If your canal is not the right shape or size, you are out of luck. Let's answer a few questions about invisible hearing aids.

What are invisible hearing aids?

Invisible hearing aids are deep fitting custom made hearing devices that sit deep within the ear canal. More often than not, the faceplate of the hearing aid cannot be seen. For this reason, they have been given the name invisible. The first manufacturer to introduce modern invisible hearing aids was Starkey, they introduced the SoundLens and it began the race across all hearing device manufacturers to introduce an invisible device. Each and every manufacturer has now introduced an invisible hearing aid option.

These hearing instrument types are called by different names by the different manufacturers, sound lens, Nano, IIC invisible in the canal or just plain invisible hearing aids. No matter the official title, they all amount to pretty much the same thing, deep canal hearing aids.

The battleground has now extended as some of the device manufacturers have now introduced wireless invisible hearing devices. Something which up to now has been technically difficult. We would expect more of the hearing brands to begin offering wireless invisible instruments over the next year. Although this market is small, while you might expect everyone to want one, not everyone is suitable.

Are invisible hearing devices suitable for everyone?

The short answer is no, not at this time, while your hearing loss obviously needs to be taken into account, the major stumbling block to suitability is normally the size and shape of your ear canal. If your ear canal is either too small, too narrow or too awkward, you won't be suitable for these devices, It is as simple as that.

Even with advancements in technology, that will probably remain the case for a few years to come. The manufacturers simply need a finite amount of space to fit all of the components in, if your canal does not offer that space, you are out of luck.

Are invisible hearing aids available on the NHS?

This is a question that we get a lot, unfortunately, the answer is no. However, there are exceptionally discreet receiver in canal hearing aids available on the NHS.

How much do invisible hearing aids cost?

Generally, they are no more expensive than a different hearing aid type from the same technology level. In other words, you generally don't pay a premium for an invisible hearing aid. I say generally, because there always may be exceptions. For instance, the Phonak Virto B Titanium (which comes in an invisible version) is slightly more expensive than a similar traditional Virto B hearing aid at the minute.

Invisible hearing aids with Bluetooth?

Again, we get asked this quite a bit, the answer is yes but no, hahaha, let me explain. There are wireless invisible hearing aids but no, they don't run on the Bluetooth connection. In the recent past, some of the hearing aid brands have released wireless invisible hearing aids.

They are wirelessly equipped and they will connect to the manufacturer's audio streaming devices. I think this is a fantastic move forward because I believe wireless hearing aids were an amazing innovation. Having said all of that, there are no Made For iPhone invisible hearing aids, there are no direct connection devices available right now.

What type of hearing loss will invisible hearing aids work with?

Generally, invisible hearing aids are suitable for moderate flattish type hearing losses. Those are generally the best types of hearing losses served by the devices. Let's take a look at other hearing loss types.

High-Frequency hearing loss and invisible hearing aids

Generally, invisible hearing aids aren't suitable for people with high-frequency hearing loss. The problem is that they have a good low-frequency hearing, so putting a device into the ear canal causes intolerable occlusion. This can be by-passed by ensuring the invisible hearing aid fits into the bony part of the ear canal. In theory, this should stop any occlusion, however, getting the device that deep in the canal can be difficult and it may be uncomfortable.

Moderate hearing loss and IIC

As I said, invisible hearing devices are ideal for flattish moderate hearing loss, there are no difficulties with occlusion and the hearing aid output is ideal for this type of loss.

Severe Hearing Loss and hidden hearing aids

In general, most hearing aid professionals would not offer invisible hearing aids to someone with a severe hearing loss. They are not ideal because they don't offer much headroom, which simply means if the hearing loss gets much worse, the hearing aid is useless. However, there are invisible hearing aids suitable for severe hearing loss from Signia.

Profound hearing Loss and Invisible in canal

There are no invisible hearing aids that are currently suitable for someone who suffers from a profound hearing loss.

The pros and cons of invisible hearing instruments

They are similar in nature to most custom hearing aids, the positioning of them may well be optimal for hearing devices. That position deep in the canal allows the outer ear and ear canal to do its job, funnel sound naturally towards the eardrum. This is probably the biggest benefit of these types of devices, however, that positioning means that all of the electronics are open to the wax an moisture in the ear canal. This means that they need a lot of care and attention from the user. They also need dehumidifying on a regular basis.

If you are prepared to take care of these hearing aids well, then I would say go ahead with them, however, you will need to take care of them to avoid electronics failures. As I said, while there are wireless invisible hearing aids, generally speaking, most invisible hearing aids are non-wireless enabled.

Completely In Canal Hearing Aids / Mini In Canal

Completely in canal or CIC hearing aids are pretty discreet devices that will go unnoticed except by the keenest eye. Up to recently, they were predominantly non-wireless, however, in just the recent past, many manufacturers have released wireless enabled CICs.

I think that this is a fantastic breakthrough; however, wireless enabled devices are slightly bigger than non-wireless CICs so you need to consider that before you go ahead if complete discretion is your objective. What is hugely interesting is that some manufacturers have managed to fit directional microphones on CICs, this again is a recent breakthrough.

Directional microphones give real assistance in noisy environments, however, this is the first time they have been on CICs so it will be interesting to see the effect they have.

Early reports indicate that they deliver better speech clarity in group and noisy situations.

Again though, directional mics make the CIC slightly larger, I believe though, that like wireless, the functionality is well worth the trade-off. Mini in canal hearing aids are all of the above with the exception that they are slightly larger, most mini in canals would come with wireless functionality and directional microphones.

Full Shell & Half Shell Hearing Aids

They are as they sound, larger custom hearing aids that sit in the concha or bowl of the ear. The half-shell basically fills half the concha and the full shell fills the whole concha. The traditional benefit of these devices has been more features, more power and physical controls like programme button and volume controls.

In the recent past with the introduction of wireless capability and more powerful solutions at CIC level, those benefits have all but become negated. However, these devices still have advantages, they usually have bigger battery sizes which allow them to work longer between changes and they are easier to handle for people with dexterity and vision problems.

The Pros & Cons of Custom Hearing Aids

Yes, you guessed it, there are most definitely advantages and disadvantages to custom hearing aids. Let's take a deeper look at what they are.

What Are The Advantages Of Custom Hearing Devices?

Discreet

The smaller devices are highly discreet and the invisible hearing aids are in fact, invisible. The larger devices are of course not as discreet.

Easy To Handle

Because the devices are all in one unit they can be easy to handle and to place in the ear especially the larger hearing aids.

What Are The Disadvantages of Custom Hearing Devices?

Receiver Issues, Microphone Issues

Like RIC / RITE devices, the receiver is placed in the ear canal, however, it is better protected than the receivers in RICs. Again this placement exposes not just the receiver but all of the electronic components including the microphones to the hostile environment that the ear.

The manufacturers take great pains to protect both the receivers and the microphones. However, unless you take good care of your hearing aids, changing your wax guards when you should and cleaning the microphones, you are looking at possible failures.

Dirt and Wax, a Nightmare for Hearing Aids

At best, wax or dirt can just block the sound outlet or microphone inlet, at worst, it can make its way into the components itself and destroy them. As we said wax and moisture is the kiss of death for electronics. The manufacturers have done a good job of protecting those sensitive components in most cases.

It is very rare for anything other than the microphone or receiver to fail, chipset failures are that rare that they are remarked upon with surprise.

In the case of custom hearing aids, if there is a failure they will have to be sent off for repair which can take a varying amount of time. If the failure is under warranty it will be repaired free of charge, if not, you will have to pay a fee. If you are having them repaired regularly, the cost adds up.

Good Clean and Care

The key to success with these hearing aid types is a good clean and care routine that involves drying. The better you take care of these hearing aids, the better they will perform. Again, I don't want to put you off this device types, they are fantastic devices and I really like them. If you are recommended this type of device just be aware of the inherent issues.

As we said, many of the hearing healthcare professionals we partner with can arrange a five-year manufacturer's warranty to cover repairs. Some may charge, some may actually offer it for free. If you are considering buying custom hearing aids, ask about an extended manufacturer's warranty.

Maybe Too Small!

Some of the custom hearing aids are very small and discreet devices, as with RIC / RITE devices, the smaller the device, the smaller the battery they use. With the smaller custom devices, the size of the hearing aid and the size of the battery can cause difficulties for people with dexterity issues. |If you have difficulty handling the hearing aids or putting the batteries in, what should be a joy can easily turn into a frustrating task. The larger custom devices are easier to handle and use larger batteries that are easier to handle.

Contra-indications To Wearing Custom Hearing Aids

As with RICs and RITE devices, there are some people who shouldn't wear these type of devices. It is pretty much the same as RICs if you have permanent perforations in your ears or you have had a mastoid operation these hearing devices aren't really for you.

The same can be said for people who suffer from wet ears or produce a large amount of earwax, either condition will cause issues for the hearing aids. Even though the power output has been increased greatly with these type of hearing aids, they still might not be suitable for your hearing loss.

If they aren't, don't let vanity win, get a hearing aid that is suitable for your hearing loss. That will translate into better hearing which will help you lead a better life.

In Finishing

Again these are great devices generally, they are quite reliable, but they do need care and attention to ensure they keep on keeping on.

Behind The Ear Hearing Aids

We Love BTEs
We love BTE hearing aids, probably the most reliable hearing devices you can buy.

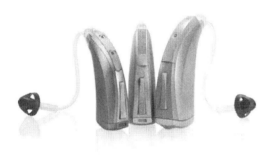

BTE Hearing Aids
Behind The Ear or BTE hearing aids have been around for a very long time. In the recent past, they have got smaller, more versatile and more powerful. Behind the ear hearing aids are self-contained units with all of the components in the case. Over recent years they have gotten much smaller than they once were. They are hugely versatile devices and they will fit nearly every hearing loss.

Normally the manufacturers will make different styles for differing losses, one for most losses from mild to severe and one usually labelled a superpower for profound hearing loss. Even the superpower devices have become quite small in comparison to the older styles. The hearing aid is connected to the ear through a coupling, in some cases, it is via a tube and ear mould, in the case of the hearing aids to the left it is with a thin tube and instant fit tip. The actual fittings are varied and usually based on hearing loss.

The Pros & Cons of BTE Hearing Aids

We are finding it hard to think of disadvantages really, but we will give it the old college try. Let's take a look at what you can expect from BTE devices.

What Are The Advantages Of BTE Hearing Devices

Fully Functional Hearing Solutions

BTE hearing aids nearly always have a full load of hardware including volume controls, programme buttons and telecoils. The telecoil is a useful addition if you want access to loop systems in public buildings like churches, conference centres, and the post office.

In fact, many taxis in London are fitted with loop systems. Even though wireless communication systems in hearing aids are now the norm, the telecoil is still a good thing to have. The only issues that occur in relation to it are how well the loop system is working or how well it has been fitted. This can affect the audio quality.

Extremely Reliable Hearing Aids

BTE hearing aids are probably the most reliable of hearing aids, they very seldom fail. Because all of the components are encased in the hearing aid and the hearing aid is worn at the back of the ear, very little or no wax or moisture can get at them.

When something goes wrong with a BTE it tends to be either the physical controls or the microphones. Nearly all of the manufacturers have introduced new types of microphone covers that almost completely enclose the microphones. So even microphone failure may be a thing of the past.

Easy To Use

BTE hearing aids tend to be easy to handle and place in the ear, so for people with dexterity or vision issues they are a good choice.

What Are The Disadvantages of BTE Hearing Devices

Haven't a Clue

We are wracking our brains here and really can't think of anything, maybe discretion? Even that isn't really true, a small BTE with a thin tube is a very discreet hearing aid to wear. It would be almost as discreet as many of the RIC / RITE devices. Okay, the larger BTEs are not the most discreet, but personally, I would always go for long-term reliability every time. A hearing aid is of no use to you if it is broke and BTEs very rarely break.

Contra-indications To Wearing BTEs

Sorry, again we are stuck for any here really.

Wireless Hearing Aids, Bluetooth Hearing Aids, What's The Difference?

Wireless Hearing Aids

I spoke earlier about wireless hearing aids, they really have made a huge difference to the function of hearing aids and the benefit provided to users. There are two different types of devices that fall under the term wireless devices. There are hearing aids that are designed to connect to a series of accessory devices supplied by a manufacturer. And there are hearing aids that are designed to connect to a series of devices supplied by a manufacturer and designed to connect directly to other devices with a Bluetooth connection.

The first category of wireless hearing aids still makes up the bulk of wireless hearing aids. They are generally great devices and the connection to their accessories is usually excellent and highly stable. The quality of the audio signal that is streamed has also increased as the systems have developed. The system from Widex is recognised for outstanding audio quality but many of the others are catching up.

The accessories for wireless hearing aids deliver a whole new level of benefit to a user. For instance, remote microphones really deliver fantastic benefit in noisy environments. These type of devices make even low technology hearing aids very powerful devices.

Made For iPhone Hearing Aids

The LiNX from GN Resound was the very first device to come onto the market from the second category. That category is generally known as Made For iPhone hearing aids. That is essentially a misnomer because they will also connect to Android Smartphones as well, just not in a direct manner; however, the name has stuck.

The LiNX was also designed to connect to GN Resound's Unite wireless accessories, which were designed to connect to phones, audio systems and TVs. What made them different from everything else at the time was that they could connect directly to an iPhone without any intermediary device. They were the very first to have this ability although they were followed quickly by the Halo from Starkey.

At the time of writing, every major hearing aid brand has released devices that will connect directly to iPhones without intermediary devices and I would expect any manufacturer who has lagged behind to do so in the near future.

The Problem with Bluetooth

All of these hearing aids are pretty outstanding devices and the fact that they connect directly without an add-on is celebrated by many users. However, they have their issues, generally, those issues are caused by Bluetooth. Although Bluetooth technology has gotten better, it is still a finicky technology which occasionally just does its own thing.

Like dropping the connection for no reason and then refusing to find the device it was just connected to. Believe me, I use Bluetooth every day for information transfer purposes and it can be infuriating. It often works exceptionally well for weeks at a time and then it doesn't, for no apparent reason.

Unfortunately, the hearing aid manufacturers can't control this, it is just a function of Bluetooth. Again, I wouldn't let this hold you back, just be aware of the problem when you are making a decision.

Rechargeable Hearing Aids

Modern Rechargeable Hearing Aids

Rechargeable hearing aids have been with us for a while; both Siemens and Hansaton have provided rechargeable hearing aids for many years. Up to now though, they have not been hugely popular. I believe this is going to change, let me first tell you why they weren't popular and then explain what will change that forever.

The main issue with rechargeable hearing aids to date has been battery technology. The batteries simply could not be trusted to power modern hearing aids and the demands of streaming audio for a full day without interruption.

Not just that, the life of rechargeable batteries tended to be about a year. After that, they did not continue to hold their charge well and needed to be replaced. For most hearing aid providers, it made little sense to recommend them to prospective users. In essence, they were perceived to be a novelty and never gained traction.

What's Changed?

The battery technology has dramatically evolved, Phonak and Signia introduced their first ever rechargeable hearing aid range that is powered by Lithium-ion batteries. Lithium-ion as a power source is more capable and a far better option for hearing aid use.

The Lithium-ion technology in the new Phonak range will deliver a full 24 hours of use on a single three-hour charge. The use time will also include streaming audio time, so if you use your hearing aids as wireless headphones for music, TV or phone connection, you will still get 24 hours of use.

Lithium-ion is also capable of far more charge-recharge cycles, however, the power pack is only expected to last three to four years which means the batteries will need to be changed during the lifetime of the hearing aids.

Phonak was, of course, the first brand to introduce the modern range of rechargeable hearing aids but they were quickly followed by Signia. The two market leaders introduced Lithium-Ion powered rechargeable hearing aids. The rest of the brands have introduced Silver-Zinc powered rechargeable hearing aids powered by the Z-Power system. There are pros and cons to both systems and I will talk about them a bit later.

Why will this change everything?

For two reasons, firstly the hearing aid industry is like an arms race, if one does something particularly innovative and well received the others will be quick to follow. Secondly and probably most importantly, consumers want it, in fact, they want it badly.

If you are an experienced user you will probably know what I mean, if you aren't, let me explain. Most experienced users have a giant size pain in their arse (Irish technical term) with disposable hearing aid batteries. They are fiddly, easy to drop and generally irritating, not just that they are also an ongoing cost.

Generally the cost is negligible; however, they are still an ongoing cost that many users resent. There is also the whole hassle of making sure you have spare batteries wherever you go. Sounds easy right? Nahhhhh, as most people will tell you, the day they forgot to pack their spare batteries was the day the hearing aids run out unexpectedly.

So we have a congruence of two states of being, Hearing aid providers are more likely to recommend rechargeable hearing aids and the market, in general, will be exceptionally receptive to them.

Why Should You Consider Rechargeable Hearing Aids?

There are many reasons why you should consider buying rechargeable hearing aids and I would like to set them out here. Generally, rechargeable hearing aid options are no more, or little more expensive than the models that use traditional hearing aid batteries, so the cost of adoption is negligible.

In the next few paragraphs, I will compare Silver-Zinc rechargeable batteries to disposable batteries. Lithium-Ion power packs are a little different in nature and need to be replaced once every three to four years. I am still unsure of the cost of replacement of Lithium-Ion power packs. So I haven't discussed them here.

Ease of Use

Rechargeable hearing aids offer real ease of use to you, no fiddling around with little batteries every few days. The size of hearing aid batteries, and in fact hearing aids themselves, can be irritating and troubling to users, especially if they have eyesight or dexterity issues. Just removing the disposable battery from the packaging can be a mini-nightmare for some people, let alone opening the battery compartment and getting the damn battery in there!

So, if you have decreased dexterity or a condition that numb the fingertips, such as arthritis, diabetic neuropathy, and Parkinson's disease well then, rechargeable hearing aids are most definitely for you. Rechargeable hearing aids are simply put into the charger at night, and in the morning they are ready for use. More than that, you don't need to remember to buy batteries, you don't need to remember to carry spares, you never run out and generally your battery won't let you down at the very worst moment.

Good for The World

Rechargeable batteries are far greener and better for the environment than disposable hearing aid batteries. With silver-zinc rechargeable batteries, you will need to replace them once a year, during a five-year time-frame, you will need 8 batteries. During the same time span, you will need on average 520 disposable batteries.

Generally Cost-Neutral

When you need to replace your rechargeable silver-zinc batteries, it will cost you on average maybe £50. So basically, apart from utility costs (electricity), a year's worth of rechargeable bliss is around fifty quid. If you shop very carefully, you could probably buy a year's worth of disposable batteries for around the same price. So the cost is probably relatively neutral. For those people who don't shop for their hearing aid batteries online, rechargeable batteries are probably a far cheaper option.

Probably only BTE and RIC for the moment

At present, it appears that this new renaissance of rechargeable will only be available in BTE and RIC models. Making custom hearing aids rechargeable is a complex operation; generally speaking, it would not be difficult to make a large custom hearing aid rechargeable (such as a full shell ITE). However, making a small ITE like a CIC rechargeable would be pretty complex.

Two manufacturers have introduced Lithium-ion rechargeable hearing aids, however, the rest have plumped for Silver-Zinc devices. Let's take a look at what is on offer.

Phonak Rechargeable Hearing Aids

Phonak kick-started this new movement with the introduction of their Audeo B-R or Belong-Rechargeable. The device is a Receiver in Canal device and it is available in their top three levels of technology. Interestingly they didn't offer it in their lowest entry level range. The device can handle several levels of receiver so it covers hearing losses from mild to profound.

They say that no matter the level of the receiver, the device will last for twenty-four hours between charges with up to eighty minutes streaming of audio wirelessly. That is pretty impressive, apparently, they have found in field trials that the devices will last for up to fifteen hours with five hours of streaming which is pretty much a full day for most users. That would mean that you would get quite a bit of answering your mobile and watching the television in as well.

The devices will run for six hours after a thirty-minute charge and a full charge takes three hours in total. They quickly followed up with the introduction of their Bolero B P-R which is a BTE powered by the same rechargeable power pack. They offer the same stats for it.

Signia Rechargeable Hearing Aids

Signia quickly joined the fray with the introduction of their Cellion Primax devices. Again, these are Receiver in Canal devices and again, they can take many levels of receivers. Signia introduced the Cellion in all of its levels of technology. They say that their devices will last 24 hours with limitless streaming. That is exceptionally impressive if it proves true (no reason to doubt them!).

The devices will run an impressive seven hours on a thirty-minute charge and a four-hour charge will fully charge them.

Oticon Rechargeable Digital Hearing Aids

Oticon was a little late to the party with their Rechargeable hearing aids offer. In an announcement reported here in April, Oticon announced the expansion of the models on the Opn range. That expansion also included a brand new rechargeable model. They too have gone down the route of the Z Power Silver Zinc technology which makes a lot of sense. Z Power systems offer real versatility and a lot of power. Although the hearing aids were announced in April, they will be available in the UK, the US and Ireland from November 2017.

Resound Rechargeable Digital Hearing Aids

Resound introduced their rechargeable hearing aids in August 2017. They have also gone down the route of using the Z Power Silver-Zinc battery technology.

Resound LiNX 3D LT61-DRWZ

The new addition to the LiNX 3D range is a completely new form factor and is similar in size if a little different from their existing LT61. The device is officially designated the LT61-DRWZ and it runs on a 312 rechargeable battery which is supplied by Z Power as is the recharging cradle technology. That means there should be plenty of power for a full day of use even if you are streaming audio and taking phone calls. The device is expected to available on the market in September. We would expect the prices to be similar to the LiNX 3D prices.

Starkey Rechargeable Digital Hearing Aids

Starkey also went for Z Power for their rechargeable hearing aids, although they have been doing some research into wireless charging of hearing aids. For now, this is the system they have gone for, but we half expect to see something different in the future.

Muse™ micro RIC 312t R

The Muse™ micro RIC 312t R is just one of the styles available on Starkey's® "made for music" hearing aid platform. The rechargeable offering is not a Lithium-ion device and nor is the power pack integrated. The power pack is actually ZPower's innovative silver-zinc battery technology. This is used with their charger to give at the very least 24 hours of use. Going with this option will allow Starkey customers to switch to normal disposable batteries if they are caught out. From what we can see the Muse micro RIC 312t R will be available in the full three levels of technology.

Starkey have just announced that they are introducing a Lithium-Ion rechargeable hearing aid this year. We will keep you updated on it as we hear more on Hearing Aid Know.

Unitron Rechargeable Digital Hearing Aids

Unitron quickly followed their stablemate Phonak (both owned by Sonova) with their own rechargeable hearing aids. However, unlike Phonak, they went for the Z Powered Silver-Zinc option. They first introduced a Receiver In Canal rechargeable option but have since followed with a Behind The Ear Option.

Moxi Fit R Hearing Aids

Smallest Rechargeable Hearing Aids Ever

Unitron introduced the Moxi Fit R rechargeable hearing aid option with the new Tempus platform. The Moxi Fit R is the smallest rechargeable hearing aid ever, the rechargeable kit can also be bought separately and be fitted to existing Moxi Fits.

Stride M-R Hearing Aids

A Rechargeable BTE

Unitron rounded out their rechargeable offering with a new rechargeable BTE, the Stride M R. It is their first ever rechargeable behind the ear hearing aid. The device runs on Silver-Zinc rechargeable batteries and has a similar charger to their Moxi devices. There is an auto on feature so when you take the hearing aids out of the charger they just come on. Something that many users welcome.

Widex Rechargeable Digital Hearing Aids

Widex were practically the last to the party with rechargeable hearing aids. They have been working on Fuel Cell technology for many years and when they make that breakthrough, it will change the powering of hearing aids forever. I say without hesitation that fuel cell technology will be a paradigm shift and I really hope Widex crack it.

For now, they have introduced a Z Power system for their popular Beyond hearing aids. The new rechargeable Beyond is named the Beyond Z and it is expected that it will be released in quarter four in the United States and Quarter 1 of 2018 everywhere else.

What Are The Pros and Cons of Rechargeable Hearing Aids?

Some people have warned people off rechargeable hearing aids for different reasons, I think they are exceptionally beneficial, but there are pros and cons, let's talk about the types and what they have to offer.

Rechargeable hearing aids have been around for a long time, however, there were never very popular because of power output. ZPower has coined the phrase one-charge-per-day standard, and it is a pretty good phrase (I wish I came up with it). In essence, the traditional rechargeable hearing aids did not meet the one-charge-per-day-standard. The power supply problem only got worse when hearing aids became wireless and more users were streaming audio.

A New Generation of Rechargeable!

A new generation of rechargeable battery technologies has arrived and it promises to make life easier for consumers. Lithium-ion and Silver-Zinc both of these technologies offer something different with different pros and cons, but the one thing they both offer is, the one-charge-per-day-standard.

Lithium-ion Rechargeable hearing aids

As I said earlier, two hearing aid brands offer Lithium-ion rechargeable hearing aids. In the case of Phonak, the power pack is a sealed, integrated system. Signia have delivered something similar, but different. The systems offer pros for safety and cons for the use case. Let me explain, Lithium-ion can be a fire risk if the battery is damaged, sealing the battery in the body of the hearing aid means that it is protected from mishandling.

However, sealing it in the case also means that it cannot be replaced by the user. Lithium-ion can be expected to deliver for between four and five years, so that means the battery pack will have to be replaced after four or five years because it will not be delivering what it should.

To do this, the hearing aids will have to be sent back to the factory and it will also have a cost attached. From what I know, Phonak at least has said that they will replace battery packs in the future as a normal repair, which means it won't be a ridiculous cost.

As I said, Signia has done it differently, their power pack is a sealed unit, however, they have designed the outer case to ensure that the power pack can be replaced in the office as opposed to the factory.

The Cons of Lithium-Ion Rechargeable Hearing Aids

- **Safety**: Lithium-ion is a poison, and hearing aids are small enough to swallow, presenting a hazard to children and pets. Lithium-ion has the potential to go on fire if damaged badly enough.

- **Sealed Case**: The fire hazard of the tech dictates that the lithium-ion battery is integrated into a sealed case. If it runs out of power while still in use, the hearing aid cannot run on a normal disposable battery but must be taken out of commission while it recharges. And when a lithium-ion battery reaches the end of its life, it can't be replaced by the user but must be swapped out by the manufacturer (Phonak devices) or the professional (Signia Devices).

- **Power Limitations**: If you stream a lot of audio (from an MP3 player or mobile phone, etc.), there's a possibility the batteries may not last the full 24-hour day. In fact, Phonak seem to think that if you stream up to about five hours, the aids will last 14 to 16 hours. This shouldn't affect most people though since 12-16 hours would be a typical day of hearing aid use.

- **Larger Footprint:** The footprint of Lithium-Ion is bigger than the other option which means bigger hearing aids.

-

The Pros of Lithium-Ion Rechargeable Hearing Aids

- **No more fiddly battery changes:** The technology ensures that you no longer have to worry about the expense of disposable hearing aid batteries, nor do you have to worry about changing them.

- **24 hours continuous use:** The technology has finally reached the one-charge-per-day standard. You should be able to get up to 24 hours use with up to **5 hours streaming.**

- **Easy charging**: Simply drop it in your charger, no hassle.

-

Silver-Zinc Systems

The primary producer of Silver-Zinc rechargeable hearing aid systems is ZPower. Originally ZPower offered a retrofit system which consisted of individually designed battery compartments and chargers for many popular hearing aid models. This allowed hearing aid users to change their current products to rechargeable hearing aids.

However, in partnership with two separate hearing aid brands, there are now two separate Silver-Zinc powered rechargeable hearing aid options. Like the lithium-ion systems, they provide power for a full day of use.

These systems are not integrated and sealed into the product, in fact, these systems are a little more forgiving than the Lithium-ion systems. If for some reason you don't get to charge your hearing aid, you can simply slip in a disposable battery. Silver-Zinc is also more stable than Lithium-Ion; it won't explode into flame when damaged.

The Cons of Silver-Zinc Rechargeable Hearing Aids

- **Once a Year Replacement**: Silver-Zinc batteries need to be replaced once a year. This represents a cost to you, however, they are cheap enough so the cost over four or five years probably balances out with the repair cost of changing a Lithium-Ion power pack.
- **Power Limitations**: This is less of a problem with Silver-Zinc because they are much more power dense. However, if you stream a lot of audio (from an MP3 player or mobile phone, etc.), there's a slight possibility the batteries may not last the full 24-hour day.
-

The Pros of Silver-Zinc Rechargeable Hearing Aids

- **No more fiddly battery changes:** The technology ensures that you no longer have to worry about the expense of disposable hearing aid batteries, nor do you have to worry about changing them except for once a year.
- **24 hours continuous use:** This technology is also one-charge-per-day standard. You should be able to get up to 24 hours use with up to **5 hours streaming.**
- **Flexibility**: Because they are removable, the rechargeable batteries can be easily replaced by standard disposable hearing aid batteries in the event of an emergency. The hearing aids can run on the disposables until they can be recharged at night. It also means that when it comes time to replace them, you can do it at home.
- **Safety**: Silver-zinc is non-flammable, non-toxic and 100% recyclable.

- **Smaller footprint**: Higher energy density means a silver zinc battery can come in a smaller package than comparable lithium-ion rechargeable batteries. This simply means smaller hearing aids.
- **Backward Compatible**: The technology is backwards compatible and it can be added as an aftermarket system.

As you can see, there is a lot to think about when it comes to rechargeable hearing aids, not least what type is right for you. Each system has its pros and cons, and I don't think you should be afraid of them. As always, we just think you should have all the knowledge you need to make an educated decision.

Hearing Aid Technology

Hearing Aid Technology Levels

Hearing aid technology levels can be confusing at best, why is one better than the other? Here is what you need to know.

Let's Talk Hearing Aid Technology Levels

Once upon a time, there were three hearing aid technology levels, what were known in the profession as low end, mid-range and high end. Then most of the hearing aid manufacturers introduced four, loosely they are called, basic, standard, advanced and premium and that is the designations I will use here for clarity.

The Life of a Hearing Aid

We hear many times that a hearing aid has a life of about five years, that isn't really quite true. What is meant by that is hearing aid technology radically moves forward every five years. Hearing aids themselves can last for over a decade with care and attention.

So if you buy one today, you may still be wearing it in ten or twelve years, the available hearing aid technology will have changed dramatically twice in that time. Doesn't mean that there is anything wrong with your hearing aid, it just means that there are things that are radically better available.

Let's take a look at those levels and what you can expect from them in general. Every couple of years a hearing aid manufacturer releases a new product range, once it was every four years but it seems to have accelerated to almost every two years in the recent past.

For clarity purposes, a product range may be referred to as a chipset, a platform or a family by differing people within the profession. Each new product range will have four levels of technology.

We said that there used to be three technology levels in hearing aids but that had changed, we kind of feel what the manufacturers have done in most cases is actually split the mid-range into two levels. A lower mid-range which is what we are calling standard and a higher mid-range which is what we are calling advanced.

Normally within each technology level, there will be every hearing aid type that they produce. For instance, Widex has introduced their new product range the Unique, the Unique product range is based on the new Unique chipset and it has four levels of technology, the 440 which is top of the range or premium technology, the 330, the 220 and the 110 which is the basic level of technology.

Each of those Widex technology levels has a full family of hearing aids including custom, BTE and RICs. Nearly every manufacturer offers hearing aid products in this manner, some use different names to mark different technology levels but most use some sort of name and numeral combination. Phonak like to confuse everyone by giving their hearing aid types different names, but at least they stick to the numeral using the number 90 for their premium top of the range devices, 70, 50 and finally 30 for their basic level.

How Hearing Aids Work

Before we launch into the different levels of technology, let's talk quickly about what hearing aids are. Hearing aids have changed dramatically over the last few decades with the advent of digital technology. At their core, hearing aids have always been made of the same four basic parts: a microphone, a processor, a receiver (the speaker), and a power source (the battery).

In simple terms, the microphone picks up the sounds and passes it to the processor. The processor enhances the signal in accordance with its programming and delivers it to the receiver which delivers the amplified signal to the ear canal.

The power source delivers the power needed to make the magic happen. The introduction of digital technology transformed hearing aids allowing manufacturers to introduce ever more powerful processors in smaller packages. In modern hearing aids, the signal picked up by the microphone is converted from analogue to digital before being processed, this allows for a much deeper manipulation and enhancement of the sound.

This manipulation is how noise reduction and other hearing aid features work. The signal is then converted back from digital to analogue before the receiver delivers the enhanced signal into the ear canal. It is nearly impossible to get an analogue hearing aid now, it is a special order, virtually all of the hearing aids manufactured in the world are now digital. Okay, let's take a look at what the tech levels are and more importantly what they can do for you.

Basic technology hearing aids

Each manufacturer has a basic level of technology, they may not call it exactly that but for clarity that is the label, it is getting. This level of technology is designed to work for people who are relatively sedentary (don't get out much).

As I have said, this might be the basic level but it will still be on the latest chipset available from the manufacturer. Basic level hearing aids are usually just that, quite basic, they will have features such as directional microphones and maybe even some noise reduction, more on both later, but generally they will be basic and they will be manually controlled.

However, that is beginning to change, Phonak has just introduced their latest Venture platform and the basic hearing aid technology the V30 is an automatic hearing aid. It is limited to only two sound situations, but that is an interesting development none the less.

Other manufacturers will follow suit in their next generation of hearing aids. This is just like an arms race when one does it, the others have to follow suit.

Lifestyle help from basic hearing aid technology

You can expect basic technology to help you in less complex sound situations. That means that you can expect to hear well in one to one conversations, even if the person is talking to you from another room (within reason, if you own a thirty bedroom mansion, all bets are off). You can also expect them to help you with small groups, family around the kitchen table for instance.

They should also help you with TV and Radio, although both can be a little difficult because of the quality of audio from different stations. Depending on the car you drive, this level of technology should also help you with understanding conversation in the car.

Well programmed basic hearing aids will help you somewhat with limited noise. If you take the time to learn coping strategies like turning your back to the noise and seating yourself in a way that minimises exposure to the noise. However, once the noise level rises, they will begin to let you down.

This is where our love of wireless accessories comes in, if you use a remote microphone accessory with a basic level of hearing aids it will really help you in noise. It will give you that extra bit of help you need to hear your companion, it will also open up other opportunities to hear better in different situations. In the car, you simply hand the remote mic to your passenger and you will be able to hear them quite clearly. Having issues with the TV? Put your remote mic down by the speaker, or use the cable that comes with it to plug into the audio out of the TV. By no means is it a replacement for higher technology hearing aids, but when you are working on a budget it can give you the extra edge you need.

Standard technology hearing aids

Again, each manufacturer has a standard level of technology which is second from the bottom. These devices are aimed at people who are a little more active. The features in these hearing aids will be slightly better than the basic features and are designed to help you hear in slightly more challenging sound situations.

This level of technology is designed for someone who is more active in their life. This level of technology has dramatically improved over the years, to give you an idea, the current hearing aids at this level would easily be as good as flagship models from five years ago.

Lifestyle help from standard hearing aid technology

You can expect all of the help that a basic hearing aid would deliver but better, and on top of that, you can expect help in group situations, small meetings, out and about at the shops and in restaurants.

Again, this is based on the noise levels present, this level isn't going to help you to hear well in a very noisy restaurant on a Saturday night, think moderate levels of background noise in most situations.

Again, wireless hearing aid accessories can make up for any difficulties in different situations and you should also consider them. We believe they are worth the extra expense in most cases.

Advanced technology hearing aids

This level of technology is ideal for active people delivering good sound quality and speech clarity in most situations they will find themselves in. This level of technology has dramatically improved in the last few years; it seems that most of the manufacturers are keeping a lot of their top end technology features in the advanced ranges.

They are dumbing them down slightly, but not much, it has been interesting to watch especially over the last year. For instance, the Widex 330 is almost as good as the 440 range and the Phonak V70 is almost as good as the V90 range. There are clear differences between them and there are valid reasons why you would choose the higher end technology but they are close nonetheless.

The main differences between this level and the next up are the binaural processing of hearing aid features. Put simply, hearing aids work exceptionally well when they make decisions as a pair, this extends to the features involved in delivering better hearing.

In the flagship models of all brands, most of the features are applied by the hearing aids in a combined and consolidated manner because of the communication between both hearing aids.

This really does deliver the best and most natural sound and clarity. Advanced technology level hearing aids may have most of the top end features, but they don't work together in that combined way, nevertheless, they are exceptional hearing aids generally.

Lifestyle help from advanced hearing aid technology

Again, you can expect all of the help you get from the two previous levels of hearing technology but better. Advanced hearing aid technology can be expected to assist you in even complex sound situations, especially if you use coping strategies well.

Usually, at this level, you can expect real help with hearing better in situations like large auditoriums, open plan buildings like churches. You should be able to hear quite well at the theatre, music should be a far better experience.

In general, speech clarity in noisier situations should be pretty good. So if you are an active individual who likes to socialise, goes to some meetings and gets out and about to social events, these may well be the hearing aids for you. We know we are boring you with our obsession with wireless accessories, but hey good honest advice remember? Yes, wireless accessories that are chosen with the situations you really want to hear in mind will help you even more.

Premium level hearing aids

This level of technology is where the hearing aid manufacturers deliver all of their very latest features. This level of technology is for people who simply have to hear well in almost every situation. They are designed to handle the most complex sound situations and deliver the best speech clarity and most natural sound.

In this level the hearing aids will truly work as a pair, deciding on how the sound is processed to deliver the very best hearing possible. The decision-making process and the application of the hearing aid features are undertaken in a binaural manner and because it uses the power of two separate processors these are always the most powerful hearing aids available (in computing power).

Lifestyle help from premium hearing aids

Pretty much what you would expect, everything that the rest can do but exceptionally better. Premium hearing aid technology is designed to deliver the very best possible hearing and speech clarity in even complex sound situations.

These type of devices are designed for active people who need to hear well everywhere. Remember though, even at this level of technology you will not be delivered super hearing, hearing aids are designed to give you the best experience with your residual level of hearing.

They are not designed to, nor can they give you back your normal hearing or better than normal hearing. Oh, and yes, wireless accessories are still an option worth thinking about even at this level.

Hearing Aid Features, What Do They Do?

Let's Talk Hearing Aid Features

Technology levels and hearing aid features are linked, the better the technology level, the better the feature that is used. The feature set of any hearing aid is dependent on the level of technology of the hearing aid and the manufacturer.

The flagship or highest technology hearing aids from each manufacturer have the best feature set available from them. First of all, when we speak about features in the profession, we are usually not talking about physical features but hearing aid algorithms or mini programmes that run on the processor.

The easiest way to understand is to compare it to a smartphone, a smartphone runs on an overall system like Google's Android or Apple's IOS, however, within that system, there are apps available to you that do different jobs.

Hearing aids and their features are not unlike that concept. Many people get a little snowed under when they try to understand features and we can understand that. Modern digital hearing aids have a ridiculous amount of different features that are designed to deliver different levels of benefit to hearing aid users.

All modern hearing aids will have some mixture of different level of features so we are going to try and investigate them and tell you in plain language what they actually do. Please forgive me in advance, I am a nerd and this stuff excites me.

What are the real world benefits of hearing aid features?

As I discuss the hearing aid features I will try and translate them into real-world benefits for you. Just explaining what they are and what they do is simply not enough. So without further blah, let's have a look.

Audible indicators in hearing aids

Right at the basics, an audible indicator informs you of some sort of change in the hearing aids you are wearing. For instance, if you change the programme, or if the volume control has changed or that your battery is running low.

In most hearing aids these tones are usually a beep or melody type sound. Widex are one of the only manufacturers that employ real speech to announce the programme that you are on and whether your battery is low.

They have even made this feature available in many world languages. This is a clear indication of why Widex is a little different to everyone else, they think clearly about the little details that would help.

They are one of the very few manufacturers to use this feature and it is available across their range of hearing aids no matter what the technology level.

What are the advantages for you?

Audible indicators allow you to know what is happening in your hearing aids at any one time, for instance, you enter your favourite restaurant and it is busy. You know that your hearing health professional has set up programme two for just this very situation, so you switch your hearing aids to it.

You hear the two audible beeps or if you are wearing a Widex it announces the programme name, and you know immediately you are at the right settings. It is still a bit loud though, so you turn down the volume a bit, the sound of the descending beeps let you know it is working. Simply put, audible indicators allow you confidence that you are using the hearing aid properly.

Listening programmes in hearing aids

Many hearing aid manufacturers offer listening programmes in their hearing aids. What they are is a differing number of pre-set listening situations that are programmed into hearing aids. Each listening programme has its settings optimised for different listening conditions/sound environments.

The different listening programmes can then be selected by the user using a switch or push button on the hearing instrument or via a remote control The listening conditions are usually set as speech, speech in noise, music and acoustic telephone.

What's the advantage to you?

Apart from the obvious one of offering better hearing in differing situations, there are other advantages. For instance, your hearing healthcare professional can make adjustments for just one situation in isolation without making global changes to how the hearing aids work.

This means that they can target changes to help you hear better in the situation you are having a problem with, without affecting the working of the hearing aids in other situations where you are doing fine. In essence, the more programmes, the better the customisation of the hearing aid for you in different situations.

For a real-world instance, you leave the house in the morning with the children in the back of the car, so you change the listening programme to the one that focuses to the back so you can hear them clearly, all though in fairness after you did it, you wish you hadn't!.

After dropping them off you have to meet your friend in the coffee shop, the shop is busy so you use the programme that has been set up for noisy environments so you can hear her clearly. You are really glad you did because she has some great news to share with you and you can hear it clearly. That is the benefit of listening programmes.

Automatic programmes in hearing aids

Many manufacturers offer different levels of automatic programmes, what they do is automatically select the optimum instrument settings without the user having to push a button or use a switch. The management systems of the hearing instruments analyse and identify the current sound environment.

The management system decided what is the best set of parameters for you to hear better in that sound situation and then automatically switches the parameters within the hearing aids to the appropriate settings. The amount of automatic programmes on any hearing aid is dependent on the manufacturer and the technology level.

What's the advantage to you?

Automatic programmes deliver real advantages, in essence, the hearing aids are always working to deliver the best possible sound quality no matter where you are. They do so seamlessly and without any input from you, which means you can just concentrate on getting on with your life.

In most manufacturers' hearing aids, these automatic programmes can also be individually altered or fine-tuned for your preference. Most hearing aid manufacturers would also offer manual listening programmes alongside their automatic function. Again this delivers the benefit that your professional can deliver the exact customised settings you need for just one situation.

Binaural synchronisation

Binaural synchronisation is something that has only recently entered the lexicon of hearing aid terms with the advent of wireless communication between hearing aids. In essence, it means that the hearing aids communicate wirelessly to ensure that the settings are synchronised.

What's the advantage to you?

It is a hugely useful feature that was introduced several years ago. At its most basic, this feature ensures that the current user settings are synchronised across the two hearing aids. So if you make a change in one hearing aid, such as the changing the listening programme or volume control setting by touching the button. It is automatically changed on the other to reflect this. This means that the two devices are always in the same programme and at the same volume level.

However, it is at its most advanced where it dramatically improves the lives of hearing aid users. Binaural synchronisation at its most advanced makes sure that every feature of the hearing aid is working in a combined manner to deliver the very best listening experience.

This really is exciting stuff (god that was so geeky!) because it is responsible for the huge advances in hearing aids in the last few years. It is also the reason why hearing aids have become more natural sounding (told you I was a nerd). When someone speaks about this technology to you, be sure to be clear exactly what it synchronises across the two hearing aids.

Binaural Compression

Again the advent of this feature was enabled because of the advances in wireless communication in hearing aids. Widex was first to introduce it in their flagship Clear hearing aids in 2009. Most of the manufacturers have followed suit in more recent times introducing the feature under differing names.

Hearing aids that use binaural compression work as a combined system to deliver enhanced sound as natural as possible. This is achieved by using both hearing aids to assess the surrounding sound environment. This information is then shared between and used by the hearing aids in a combined manner. This mass of information allows the hearing aids to make decisions on sound output as a true pair or system.

What's the advantage to you?

The system uses natural sound cues such as temporal effects (time differences in sound) and the head shadow effect (differences in sound from one ear to the other) to assess exactly what is going on in the sound environment. It then reproduces those sound cues in the enhanced sound you receive to deliver the most natural sound experience.

All of this happens instantaneously without time lag. Because the natural sound cues are preserved, your brain gets the optimum information possible in order that it can do, what it does naturally. Remember, the ears just carry sound, it is the brain that makes sense of what you are actually hearing.

I really think that this is the most exciting feature that has been released in recent times. As this feature evolves, it will make hearing aids better and better, achieving benefits for most users that were unimaginable even a few short years ago.

Compression channels

Compression channels have kind of fallen out of favour in the recent past as a sexy talked about feature because of two reasons. The first is that they are actually hard to explain without resorting to gobbledygook and the second being that sexier more understandable features have come about.

However, they are still fantastic features and it is worth me trying to explain what they are. Okay, this is pretty technical stuff, but I will give it a go to make it intelligible.

Compression channels are designed to change how different frequencies of sound are amplified. Compression channels are divided into a number of channels that are used to restrict or change differing levels of amplification within one sound frequency.

For instance, you may have problems hearing sounds below 40dB in one channel. However, the amount of amplification we need to deliver to you to hear those sounds clearly is radically different to the amount of amplification that we may have to add to a sound of 65 dB. Compression channels allow us to add varying levels of amplification to varying volume of sounds.

The feature is used to instruct the hearing aid to amplify or reduce the range of noises that you hear. This feature simply allows us to customise the hearing aids to your hearing loss in a better manner. Some hearing aids have more channels/bands than others.

What's the advantage to you?
Simply a better-customised hearing aid which is the foundation that everything else relies upon.

Data logging

Data logging is a feature which records different sets of information during the hearing aid's use. Most hearing aid manufacturers offer data logging of one type or other with differing levels of data captured. This information is available to be analysed by the hearing professional when they connect to the hearing aids. This type of information allows a professional a deeper understanding of your experiences.

What's the advantage to you?
It can assist in the fine-tuning of the aid to your preferences. The data recorded includes the hours of use, the types of listening environments you were in, the listening programmes you used and any volume control changes during that period.

Data logging delivers information that helps the hearing professional to programme the hearing aid to your specific requirements. Anything that helps the programming of your hearing aids to better suit you has to be seen as a good thing.

Feedback cancellation in hearing aids

Feedback is the horrible whistling that is most associated with older hearing aids and used to be one of the biggest complaints of hearing aid users. Feedback is caused by amplified sound being re-processed, in other words, sound emitted from the receiver (speaker) is re-processed through the hearing aids and it shrieks. This is exactly the same thing that happens when a microphone is put too close to a speaker.

The underlying cause of feedback is the escape of sound from the ear canal. There are many reasons for that, it can be due to a poor fitting of an ear mould or in-ear hearing aid, which allows amplified sound to escape.

Earwax blockage is another frequent culprit for hearing aid feedback. Another cause of feedback is the close proximity of the hearing aids to something, for instance, if you place anything over your ear, a hand or hat or a person hugging you.

Feedback cancellation is a feature that identifies and stops feedback, how it does it changes from manufacturer to manufacturer and within technology levels. Suffice to say, each feature identifies the feedback and which frequency or frequencies it is occurring in.

It then removes the feedback from the signal and stops the whistling. Different features do this in different ways, I won't bore you with the technical details, but if you really want to know, drop us a line and we can explain.

What's the advantage to you?

Simply put, your hearing aid doesn't whistle, you don't get embarrassed and your hearing aids work better.

Adaptive feedback cancellation

This is feedback cancellation on steroids, it is able to automatically adapt its speed of operation to improve its performance, and for example, it can change how it works when you are using a telephone, listening to music and suddenly hear alarm beeps.

The telephone needs strong feedback cancellation, the music situation needs very little feedback cancellation because musical notes can sound like feedback and alarm beeps is a similar concept.

Directional microphones

Directional microphones completely changed how hearing aid users can hear in noise. Directional microphone features use the sound information supplied by two microphones, to allow the computer brain of the hearing aid to identify sound that is coming from the rear and sound that is coming from the front.

This allows the processor to reduce the level of sound coming from the rear and concentrate on the sound coming from the front. Modern directional microphone features actually enable you to change the direction of hearing as you require. You can change the focus of the hearing aids from all-around sound to being more focused on a single person or object to the front side or rear.

What's the advantage to you?
Simply put, directional microphones are a proven method for hearing well in noise. So they are an invaluable feature for you to have.

Adaptive directional microphones

Yes, you guessed it, directional microphones on steroids! This feature allows the null of the directional microphones to adapt, the null is where the noise source is. So the microphones detect the location of the strongest noise source and adapt the sound to reduce your perception of that noise.

If the noise source moves, the system adapts to keep that noise source reduced. Most of the modern adaptive systems work in more than one frequency band, meaning that they can help to reduce your perception of several different noises at one time, even if they are all moving at different positions once they are at differing frequencies.

What is the advantage to you?
Bigger, better-proven method to help you hear in noisy environments!

Automatic directional microphones

This is a feature that just automates the directional microphones completely, it allows the processor to select how it will use the directional microphones according to the sound situation you are in. In a quiet situation, they will operate in an Omni-directional mode (taking in sound from all around) and directional mode or adaptive directional mode if available when a noise source is introduced.

What's the benefit to you?
Complete automation of what is an outstanding feature, you get to hear well in every situation without any input. It just happens automatically. each manufacturer has its own flavour of directionality, where possible we will always explain what it is clearly on our website.

Frequency bands in hearing aids

Again, like compression bands or channels this one is a little bit in depth. Frequencies, as we will discuss them here, are the way that sound is split. The total frequency range of a hearing instrument is divided into a number of bands or channels in which the gain that is provided can be customised to your hearing loss.

A quick but worthwhile side note here, the frequency bandwidth of hearing aids can be very different. What that means is that the number of sound frequencies that a hearing aid can process can be very different from manufacturer to manufacturer.

Some hearing aids can only process sound frequencies between 200 Hz and 6 KHz; others can process between 100 Hz to 11.5 KHz. Why is this important? I hear you ask, while human speech is normally between 200 Hz and 4 to 6 kHz, for the full and rich enjoyment of music, a much wider bandwidth is more desirable. Hence, if you are an audiophile, you might well appreciate the wider bandwidth.

Back to frequency bands, each manufacturer is different, some hearing aid manufacturers call them bands and some call them channels and some manufacturers offer more than others. The bands allow your professional to programme the hearing aid in a more customised way for your hearing loss. The more frequency bands that the aid has, the finer the programme can be, so you end up with crisper, clearer hearing.

Most features of hearing aids work within the bands, so the more bands there are in the instrument the more bands that the features in the hearing aid work across. How many bands are best? There is a lot of debate about that, but it is generally agreed that any amount between fifteen and twenty is optimal, that's why you will find most flagship hearing aids have numbers of channels or bands in that range.

For instance, Widex flagship hearing aids have fifteen channels, however, GN Resound believe have seventeen channels.

What's the advantage to you?

The more frequency channels or bands hearing aids have the better, although after twenty the benefit starts to fade. The more channels or bands, the better the customisation and the better experience that other hearing aid features will supply. Simply meaning that you will receive optimal benefit from your hearing aids.

Hearing aid noise reduction

This is probably the feature that drives most interest, it is often discussed as a feature that makes speech clearer in noise. Generally, it actually doesn't quite do that exactly. Only one manufacturer, Widex, have actually ever produced a noise reduction feature that affects the signal to noise ratio.

Signal to noise ratio or SNR to geeks like me is used to measure the ratio of signal (speech) to noise. So the actual measure of any feature that helps you to understand speech should be SNR. What most noise reduction features actually do is to reduce the amplification of non-speech sounds in an effort to allow a better understanding of speech sounds.

This tactic makes it more comfortable for a user in noisy conditions by reducing the background noise, for example in traffic noise in the street, a busy pub or restaurant. There is a lot of evidence that this reduces fatigue, reduces the amount of concentration you have to have and therefore actually does help you hear speech a little clearer.

As with all features, not all noise reduction is the same and the more high-end technology has better strategies to deal with noise.

What's the advantage for you?
A better chance for you to understand speech in noisier environments, in combination with a good directional microphone system it will dramatically improve your experience.

Speech enhancement
Speech enhancement is another feature designed to help you hear speech clearly in noise. It is used in combination with noise reduction to better help you to hear those important speech sounds. The processor in the hearing aids identifies speech signals and enhances or amplifies them. It analyses sound signals and, where most noisy maximises the speech signal.

What's the advantage for you?
In combination with noise reduction and directional microphones, it allows you the best opportunity to hear speech in noisy sound situations.

Transient noise reduction
This is simply a noise reduction feature that concentrates on identifying and suppressing impact or sudden sounds, such as shutting doors, clattering dishes and glass breaking. The feature is designed to do it without affecting the speech clarity. It is known by many names across different hearing aid manufacturers.

No matter what it is called, it allows the hearing aid to process sudden or loud noises in a more comfortable way for the user.

What's the benefit for you?

A much more comfortable listening experience for you as you go about your daily life.

Wind noise reduction

It is exactly what it sounds like, it is a noise reduction system that reduces the sound of wind cavitation on the hearing aid microphones. This feature is particularly useful for people who like to be in the outdoors. So if you are a golfer or a hiker, it is something that you should consider.

What's the benefit for you?

It will make it much easier for you to tolerate being outdoors if you are an outdoorsy type, golf and such things, it is an invaluable feature.

I think this covers the most obvious features available, as I said, different manufacturers call the features different things. But at their core, they are the features that I have discussed here. If I have missed something that you would like to know about, drop us a line on Hearing Aid Know and we will answer your questions.

Over The Counter Hearing Aids, What Will They Mean

Over the Counter Hearing Aids

I spoke about this on Hearing Aid Know last year, but I think it is worth covering here. I think that Over the Counter hearing aids will become a bigger feature of the hard of hearing world over the next few years. There has been growing speculation in relation to Over the Counter (OTC) hearing aids being made legal in the United States and finally in 2017 instructions were passed to the FDA to regulate for such devices.

The PCAST (PRESIDENT'S COUNCIL OF ADVISORS ON SCIENCE AND TECHNOLOGY) Report in relation to hearing technology in October 2015 recommended a major change to the laws governing the supply and provision of hearing aids. One of the recommendations it made was in relation to the hearing aid medical waiver. This has now happened, what does it mean for OTC hearing aids and more importantly, what will it mean for consumers? Let's look at the background.

A Greedy Monopoly

For many years hearing aid advocate organisations in the States have been calling for changes to the rules governing hearing aid provision. The main reason for these calls has been the assumption that the high price of hearing aids has been the main block to adoption of them by the multitude of people who need them. I personally don't necessarily subscribe to that argument, I know that cost is an issue, however, I don't feel it is the general impediment that it has been painted to be.

In this debate both the manufacturers of hearing aids and the providers of hearing aids have been painted as greedy and supporting a monopoly. Unfortunately, some of the hearing provider's representative organisations have not helped themselves with ridiculous paternalistic statements that seem to have been purposefully designed to irritate people.

Are We Greedy?

I know I am not; I would have to say the bulk of people who I know within the profession are not either. I charge for my time and service and then I deliver that time and service as I am sure many others do. The focus in this debate has been on the hearing aid as a product, it has not been on how that product is delivered and maintained. The problem though is that no matter what I say, it just looks like I am defending a monopoly.

On the 7th of December, the FDA issued the "Immediately in Effect Guidance Document: Conditions for Sale for Air-Conduction Hearing Aids," which effectively ends federal enforcement of the hearing aid medical waiver. What does that mean for the consumer? The hearing aid medical waiver is a waiver that may be signed in lieu of having the required pre-hearing-aid-purchase medical evaluation. The wording of the original federal regulation can be seen here (21CFR801.421). In essence, it removes the need for a customer over the age of eighteen to get a medical evaluation of their hearing before deciding on hearing aids.

The FDA announcement does not change any rules regarding over-the-counter (OTC) hearing aids, but it did address them. "FDA does intend to consider and address those recommendations in the future as appropriate, including those regarding a regulatory framework for hearing aids that can be sold directly OTC to consumers, without the requirement for consultation with a credentialed dispenser. FDA intends to solicit additional public input from stakeholders before adopting such an approach".

In the press release " the FDA Commissioner Robert Califf, M.D. was quoted as saying "Today's actions are an example of the FDA considering flexible approaches to regulation that encourage innovation in areas of rapid scientific progress, The guidance will support consumer access to most hearing aids while the FDA takes the steps necessary to propose to modify our regulations to create a category of OTC hearing aids that could help many Americans improve their quality of life through better hearing." I think that was taken as a clear sign that with time, OTC hearing aids will become a reality.

For many years I have spoken with hearing aid advocates around the world, advocates like Steve my co-author Hearing Aid Know. Nearly all of them have been demanding more power over their hearing aids, the ability to make fine tuning changes themselves. I have always supported that idea, why shouldn't we make their hearing care inclusive? One thing that has always struck me during these conversations is that what they called for was inclusion in the process not the exclusion of the professional. Even the most strident and independent of Advocates want the ability to consult with a professional.

Would it surprise you to find out that I would support this type of hearing devices? Because I would.

You may find it surprising but I think these types of devices are a good thing, not a bad thing. However, they will only be a good thing if certain criteria are met. The devices will need to be fitted to your loss in some way, so there needs to be some way of testing your needs either built into the device or accompanying the device. Any testing procedure needs to be able to flag referable conditions, this is an imperative.

In my career, I have identified four people with cancer through a hearing test. I, of course, did not make that diagnosis; I simply undertook the hearing test and referred them for further investigation because I was deeply un-happy with the results. Four people who went on to have lifesaving treatment because of a hearing test.

Hearing loss is more often than not run of the mill hearing loss; however, sometimes it is not. Sometimes it is a sign of some underlying nefarious condition that needs treatment. This is what scares me and other people within the profession. However, good technology can probably ensure that is not an issue. I think it is incumbent upon the FDA and any other regulatory body to ensure some sort of strong regulations are in place in relation to this.

What will it Mean For You

When the new legislation is brought forward to legalise the sale of OTC hearing aids it will mean that you can go to your local point of sale and buy an OTC hearing aid just like you would buy any electronic device. You will then have to work out how to fit it and use it flying solo as it were. I think that this type of solution will not be a fit for everyone and I don't think the devices will be any better than very basic hearing aids.

Not for Everyone

Even within the traditional hearing aid manufacturers, there has been a push towards giving users more control over the hearing devices. However, not every user is interested in having the control, in fact, many want something that they put on and never have to think about.

OTC devices will be ideal for some and not for others. There was a recent small-scale study on the efficacy of self-fitted hearing aids that I reported on. The conclusions were very interesting, although the study was small, it has added some weight to the call for further study. Its conclusions were as follows

"While limited, the data suggest that self-fitting aids may provide satisfactory benefit and performance to those who can manage the self-fitting process. Our findings show that at least one currently available self-fitting product is comparable to those measured with professionally dispensed hearing aids"

What they said, in essence, was that when people were "able to manage" it seemed that self-fitting may not be a bad thing. By able to manage, they meant technically aware and able, people who were au fait or familiar with technology.

In this context, I think that OTC hearing aids will be very similar, they will be ideal for people who can manage them. However, they might not be ideal for everyone. I believe they will be similar in concept to many of the hearing aids that are already offered as internet sales.

The Freedom to Mess it up

These devices will also give you the freedom to make a mess of your hearing, this is another factor that the FDA needs to consider. It needs to ensure that you can't make your hearing worse through use of these devices. Again, I think technology can help here but it is an issue that needs to be raised. In essence, for these devices to be safe to use, users will need some education in relation to making them safe to use.

I have talked to others within the business for some time about adopting low-cost devices that were sold on an over the counter type basis. I would adopt these types of devices, I would insist that I did a work up on your hearing or you had a workup done by someone I trust (this is to protect both you and me). I would then sell you the device for you to do with it what you wanted.

If you wanted support or help other than warranty issue I would charge you for it. I think that is fair, my time is worth money, you would not expect to attend any other professional for consultation for free, so why would you expect to do so with me? I think that this may well be the future model; I don't think the traditional model will die quite yet, I think this new model will probably run in tandem with the traditional model.

What about Traditional Manufacturers?

What will the traditional hearing aid manufacturers do when OTC comes to pass? I don't know, I can't speak for them but I think they will have to re-assess their own ideas about provision channels. I don't and would not hold that against them, it is just the way of the world and of business.

I know some of them wouldn't be eager to become involved, however, business is like an arms race, when one ups the game, the others must do so to survive. As well as that, many of the hearing aid manufacturers are public companies, their management teams will need to make decisions based on their shareholders best interests.

It would be my feeling that they will take a watching brief on the market and then decide to enter it.

What Will Be Your Experience?

I think that really depends on who makes the devices, hearing aids are a specialist electronic device. Hearing aid manufacturers are producing good devices based on years of experience and research and design. New entrants to the market don't necessarily have that experience or the algorithms that make everything work.

A hearing aid is not just a simple amplifier; it does so much more than amplify sound. So it will be interesting to see what the first OTC hearing aids are like in relation to efficacy. If the traditional manufacturers become involved in this market it will mean that there will be some pretty good devices available.

Care of the Devices

Any buyer of these types of devices will have to actually take care of them, any vendor of the device will have to consider the failure of the receiver. It is pretty simple, earwax and moisture kill receivers (the speaker part) and any seller of the devices will have to be aware of that.

At the moment, traditional hearing aid manufacturers accept when your negligence (and that is often what it is) kills one of their receivers during the warranty period. They simply replace them, even when they are gummed up with ear wax.

How will that work with over the counter hearing aids? Will they continue to replace the receiver even when you have been responsible for its failure? I mean at the moment, the hearing aid manufacturers don't actually have to, but they do it. What will OTC manufacturers do?

Making the Right Choice

I try to be very careful about the recommendation I make, I try to take into account lifestyle, personal and ear canal conditions. For instance, if you are active, able and a bit tech smart, I will easily consider a RIC device or a custom hearing aid device for you. I would base that on the fact that you can easily take care of the device, ensuring that it is maintained in order that the receiver won't fail.

If however, I think that the maintenance of the hearing aid may be a problem, or if in fact, the ear canal is just too hostile (excess ear wax or moisture) I would nearly always recommend a BTE. As a purchaser of an OTC device, how are you to make the decision on that, if you make the wrong decision, what are you going to do?

Freedom

It is obvious that there are a lot of questions to answer, however I think that OTC hearing aids will bring freedom of choice, I think that can be a good thing and a bad thing. I don't think consumers are stupid, generally, well most of them. I think that delivering freedom of choice will allow people to adopt amplification earlier. Will allow them to test the water as it were, to understand what amplification can deliver to their life. That has to be a good thing.

Cleaning & Caring For Your Hearing Aids

Clean and Care of Hearing Aids

Hearing aids are small, electronic devices that operate in conditions that are both warm and damp. Conditions that most electronics don't like. After making a large investment in being able to hear better, it makes a lot of sense for you to keep them in the best shape possible by cleaning and maintaining them at home.

The hearing aid manufacturers take great efforts to ensure your hearing aid will keep on keeping on. However, if you don't do your part, those hearing aids will fail. In many cases, a failure may well end up needing to be sent away for repair.

This could leave you without your hearing aid for up to two weeks depending on how busy the repair centres are. This is a major hassle, in my experience people who have become used to better hearing with their hearing aids hate to be without them. It really upsets them, so the key is to maintain your hearing aids as much as possible to avoid any hassle.

Avoid hearing aid repairs

Hearing aids do fail, it is a fact of life, electronic components can fail, and they certainly will with age and constant use. But you can take steps to avoid that failure for as long as possible. Those steps should be incorporated into a good daily clean and care routine.

Most of the time I was in Practice, the failures I saw were a receiver (loudspeaker part) or microphone failures. It was exceptionally rare to see anything else within a hearing aid fail. Both of these components are the most exposed in every hearing aid.

They are the components that need daily attention. Some hearing aid types are more prone to possible failure than others. For instance, in the ear hearing aids and receiver in the canal hearing aids have a greater failure rate than behind the ear hearing aids.

Hearing Aid care and maintenance

So let's get to the meat, how you can best take care of your aids, I will discuss each type of aid and each step that needs to be taken. If I miss anything, let me know. Likewise, if you have some good tips yourself, don't hesitate to contact us. Before we move on here is some quick tips for hearing aid nirvana:

Follow a daily routine

Clean the hearing aids giving attention to the receivers and microphones

Dry out your hearing aids

Quick tip:

Never use alcohol, solvents or cleaning agents on your hearing aids. Special care products for cleaning like hearing aid wipes and sprays are available and should be used.

Cleaning of hearing aids and cleaning tools

You should clean your hearing aid every day, every manufacturer supplies a cleaning kit with their hearing aids.

It will usually include a wax brush, a wax pick and a cloth. These tools are designed to help you care for your aids and using them properly will help to keep your hearing aids going.

Hearing aid manufacturers have also designed filters to protect receivers in the case of RIC and ITE hearing aids.

You will also get at least one pack of these with your hearing aids. **Use Them,** the proper use of wax filters (sometimes called wax caps) will protect your receiver and keep it going longer.

Quick Tip:

Earwax & moisture kills hearing aids, wax guards are there for a reason, use them!

The biggest cause of failure is wax and moisture getting into the receivers or the microphones of hearing aids. If you change your wax guards when they need to be changed you can avoid much of this problem.

When do wax guards need to be changed?

I am sorry, but the honest answer is how long is a piece of string? Each person is different, I have seen Patients who only needed to replace their wax guards once every six months, I have seen other Patients that needed to change them every month.

It depends on wax production in the ear canal. Generally as a rule of thumb, if your wax guard is full of wax that doesn't fall out when brushed, it is time to replace it. If you don't, that wax will eventually make it into the sound tube and then the receiver.

Cleaning and maintenance of an ITE and RIC hearing aid

ITE hearing aids, in particular, need daily attention, as do RIC hearing aids. The reason for this is that the receiver lives in the ear in both devices. As I said earlier, these devices are equipped with wax guards that you need to pay special attention to. So let's break down the steps you need to take and when you should take them:

Quick tip:

Many people try to clean their aid at the end of the day, I always recommended doing it in the morning after drying it overnight. That way the wax is dry and easier to remove.

1. Place your hearing aids in a drying device at the end of the day, this will allow moisture to be removed from both the electronics and any wax or debris gathered on the aid.

2. The next morning, have a good look at the microphone inlets and the receiver end of the hearing aids. Get yourself a magnifying glass if you need to for this. The details and placement of these areas will be in your owner's manual or your hearing professional will show you.

3. Concentrate on cleaning the receiver and microphone ports using the soft-bristle brush that came with the cleaning kit. When you do it in the morning, the wax should be dried out and easy to move especially after drying out overnight.

4. To clean off built-up wax, hold the hearing aid and gently clean the openings with the wax brush. The dried debris should be loose enough to be cleaned away.

5. If there is still wax in the ports that has not been dislodged, you can use your wax pick (again, usually included in your cleaning kit) to clear more stubborn deposits out of the ports. Be careful here, don't jab the pick in, just use it gently.

6. Check your battery compartment and the battery contacts for wax or debris, if there is any brush it off.

7. Finish by wiping the entire hearing aid with the cloth provided. This will remove leftover debris from the hearing aid.

8. Assess your wax guard, if it looks like it needs changing, change it out. If you change your wax guard when needed it will go a long way towards reducing failures.

9. Lastly, give your hearing aids a good visual once-over, with ITEs, check the casing and any joins for any signs of cracks or issues. With RIC devices check the receiver wire, make sure there are no kinks or twists that may lead to the failure of the wire.

10.

Cleaning & Maintenance of BTE hearing aids

BTE hearing aids are much harder to kill, however, you still need to clean and maintain them. Drying them is as important as it is for ITE and RIC aids. The maintenance is similar but different. So let's break down the steps you need to take and when you should take them:

Quick tip:

Drying is as important for BTEs as any other hearing aid, especially the tubes.

1. Place your hearing aids in a drying device at the end of the day, this will allow moisture to be removed from both the electronics and any wax or debris gathered on the aid.

2. Occasionally when needed, remove the ear mould and tube (if you have one) from the hook and clean it with soapy water. If your BTE has a thin tube, remove the thin tube and use the supplied wire (like a hair-thin pipe cleaner) to push through the tube. This will remove any debris.

3. Use an air blower to force water out of the tube and then place the tubing in the drying kit with your hearing aid to dry overnight.

4. The next morning, have a good look at the microphone inlets of the hearing aids. again a magnifying glass can be helpful. The details and placement of these areas will be in your owner's manual or your hearing professional will show you.

5. Concentrate on cleaning around the microphone ports and any other user controls like programme buttons or volume controls. Use the soft-bristle brush that came with the cleaning kit. Again, doing this in the morning is the ideal time, the wax should be dried out and easy to move especially after drying out overnight.

6. To clean off built-up wax, hold the hearing aid and gently clean it with the wax brush. The dried debris should be loose enough to be cleaned away.

7. If there is still wax in the ports that hasn't been dislodged, you can use your wax pick (again, usually included in your cleaning kit) to clear more stubborn deposits. Be careful here, don't jab the pick in, just use it gently.

8. Check your battery compartment and the battery contacts for wax or debris, if there is any brush it off.

9. Finish by wiping the entire hearing aid with the cloth provided. This will remove leftover debris from the hearing aids.

10. Lastly, give your hearing aids a good visual once-over, check the casing and any joins for any signs of cracks or issues.

11.

Drying out hearing aids

I have spoken several times about drying out your hearing aids in this section, I should explain the process and what you can use to do it.

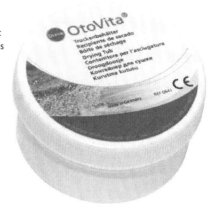

Hearing aid dryers

Hearing aid drying equipment comes in all shapes and sizes from the very cheap to moderately expensive.

It is one of the single most important investments you will make if you buy a hearing aid. Moisture build up in hearing aids cause real issues and failures and it is generally easy to avoid.

Hearing aid drying cups and tablets

Probably the simplest and cheapest form of hearing aid drying available but still very effective. It is simply a jar/cup with a sealable lid to which you drop a drying tablet into. Every night you screw the lid off, drop your hearing aids in and seal it.

The tablets are designed to suck moisture out of the air and your hearing aids. In the morning, take your hearing aids out (don't forget to seal the lid again) and voila, dry hearing aids. It is a simple process, easy to do and will save you real money in repair costs, so why wouldn't you do it?

Electronic hearing aid dryers

Yes, you guessed it, hearing aid dryers you plug in. They come with different functionality, some will still use drying tablets or bricks, and some don't. Some will dry your hearing aids and disinfect them using UV light, some won't. Many of them are designed to be portable, so you can bring them with you on trips.

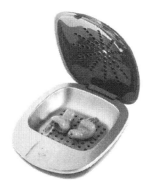

Widex introduced a drying station late last year; they call it the Dry N Go. It is a portable electronic drying and disinfecting station. You can see it to the right. There are several available on the market though.

If you follow a good clean and care routine, your hearing aids will function better for longer. Hearing aid repairs are expensive enough, so take care to avoid them with some simple maintenance.

In Finishing

I like helping people; it is actually one of my things. Don't think this is just some selfless altruistic streak. There is some of that involved but I really get a buzz knowing I helped someone. So it isn't exactly unselfish.

I would ask you to do me a great favour, if you have found this book to be of real use to you, I would ask you to give it a favourable review where you have bought it. Your reviews are important; they give the next person looking for information the confidence to buy the book.

I have covered much here and I hope I have made it clear and easy to read, however, if I have not, or if you are looking for more information, don't hesitate to contact us with your questions on Hearing Aid Know.

Printed in Poland
by Amazon Fulfillment
Poland Sp. z o.o., Wrocław